DIAGNOSTIC PICTURE TESTS IN
DERMATOLOGY

G.M. Levene MB, FRCP
Consultant Dermatologist, St John's Hospital for
Diseases of the Skin, London
and Bloomsbury Skin Unit, Middlesex Hospital, London

S.K. Goolamali MD, FRCP
Consultant Dermatologist
Central Middlesex Hospital, London
and Northwick Park Hospital
and Clinical Research Centre, Harrow, Middlesex

Wolfe Medical Publications Ltd

Titles in this series, published or being developed, include:

This Edition is produced for the Schering Corporation,
Kenilworth, New Jersey and published by
The P. W. Clinical Library
P. W. Communications International
400 Plaza Drive
Secaucus N.J. 07094
in association with Wolfe Medical Publications
London, UK

Copyright © G. M. Levene & S. K. Goolamali, 1986
Published by Wolfe Medical Publications Ltd, 1986
Printed by W. S. Cowell Ltd, Ipswich, England
ISBN 0 7234 0910 2

Schering

Schering Laboratories

Schering-Plough Corporation
2000 Galloping Hill Road
Kenilworth, New Jersey 07033
Telephone (201) 298-4000

Dear Doctor:

Schering Corporation is pleased to present you with this special edition of Diagnostic Picture Tests in Dermatology. An informative compilation of photographs depicting both common and rare dermatologic diseases, this book also includes questions that will help you test your diagnostic skills. In addition, answers to the questions are provided.

When the diagnosis is tinea cruris, corporis or pedis, the answer is LOTRISONE® brand of clotrimazole, USP and betamethasone dipropionate, USP Cream. Dual-action LOTRISONE® relieves inflammatory symptoms, such as itching and burning, while it achieves mycologic cure[*] in topical fungal infections. That's why dual-action LOTRISONE® can be so important in your practice.

Please see accompanying full prescribing information.

Sincerely,

Domenic G. Iezzoni, M.D.
Director, Medical Services

[*] A mycologic cure consists of negative cultures at the end of treatment and two weeks posttreatment.

Acknowledgements

We wish to thank Churchill Livingstone, Longman Group, for permission to reproduce illustrations 11, 12, 15, 31, 32, 60, 96 and 100 which appeared in 'Dermatology Revision', 1984, by S.K. Goolamali. We thank also Dr L. Hodge for illustration 44 and Dr M. Muhlemann for illustration 69.

We much appreciate the help given to us by Mr R.R. Phillips, Department of Medical Photography and Illustration, Middlesex Hospital, London and by Mr S. Robertson, Department of Medical Illustration, Institute of Dermatology, St John's Hospital for Diseases of the Skin, London.

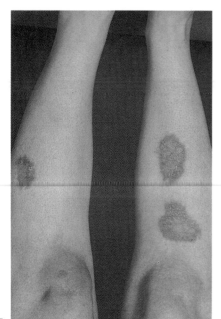

1 A 27-year-old dressmaker presented with a fleshy lesion on her index finger. No history of trauma but gentle palpation of the growth resulted in profuse bleeding.

(a) What is the lesion?
(b) What should be considered in the differential diagnosis?
(c) How would you treat it?

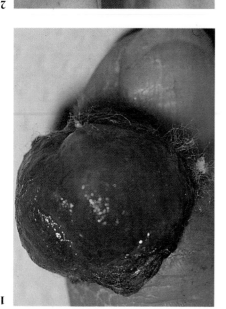

2 A 22-year-old female professional athlete developed inexplicable episodes of leg cramp, associated with nocturia which she thought was caused by increased water consumption. The legs showed the plaques illustrated.

(a) What is the skin condition?
(b) What may complicate it?
(c) Name three other skin disorders which show a predilection for the shins.

3 A 66-year-old man pre-
sented with tense dome-
shaped bullae over the knee,
thighs, forearms and umbilicus. Laboratory investigations
showed a leucocytosis, an
ESR of 14mm/hr with normal
liver function tests. Chest
X-ray showed no abnormality.
(a) What is the most likely
diagnosis?
(b) How would you confirm
it?
(c) Name 6 other blistering
diseases.

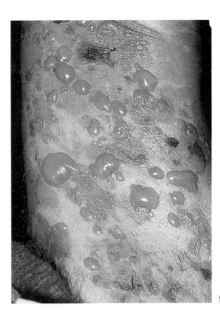

3

4 A middle-aged housewife
presented to her dentist with
mouth ulceration which had
persisted for several weeks,
despite proprietary measures.
She developed a widespread
eruption with blisters which
broke easily, leaving large
denuded areas of skin as
shown.
(a) What is the condition?
(b) What treatment is usually
prescribed?

5 Unilateral painful vesicular eruption affecting the right lower limb.
(a) What is the diagnosis?
(b) Which area of the body is most commonly affected?
(c) Name 3 complications of the disease.

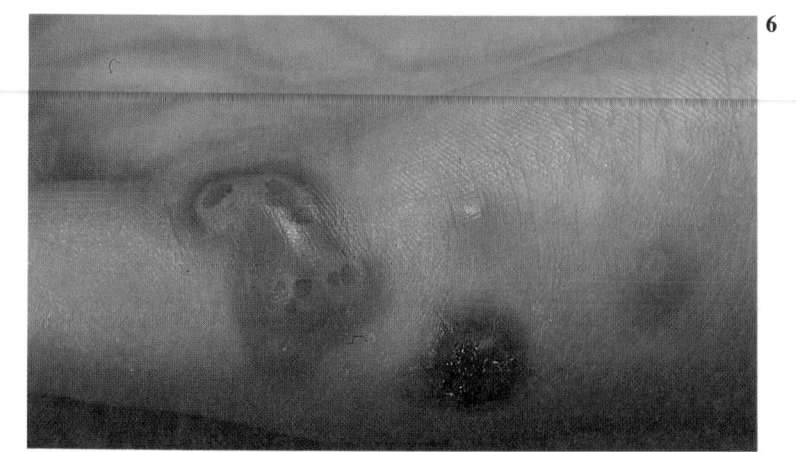

6 A physiotherapist who had suffered an abrasion over the thenar eminence of the right hand subsequently developed a vesicular eruption at the site of trauma.
(a) What is the most likely cause of the eruption?
(b) How may it have been acquired?
(c) How can you prove the diagnosis?

7 A 9-year-old girl developed severe oral ulceration with crusting of the lips and genital lesions after what her mother described as a 'heavy' cold.

(a) What is the diagnosis?
(b) What else may be involved?
(c) What may cause it?

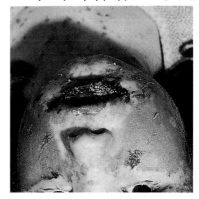

8 A 49-year-old schoolteacher became aware of a painless lesion on the scalp which grew and ulcerated over six weeks. Various topical measures had been unsuccessful. She had undergone a mastectomy three years previously.

(a) What is the lesion?
(b) How would you confirm the diagnosis?
(c) What should be considered in the differential diagnosis?

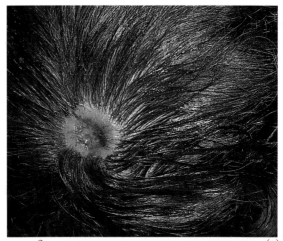

8

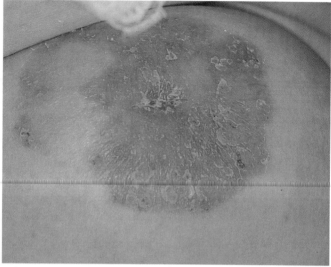

9 Photographer with pruritic, purplish, polygonal papules which heal with pigmentation.

(a) What is the diagnosis?

(b) Which drugs may cause a similar eruption.

10 Unilateral non-pruritic breast eruption. No improvement with topical corticosteroids, antibiotics or antifungals.

(a) What is the diagnosis?

(b) What important physical sign differentiates it from eczema?

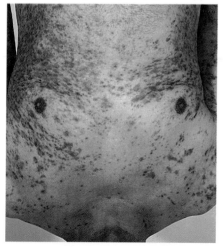

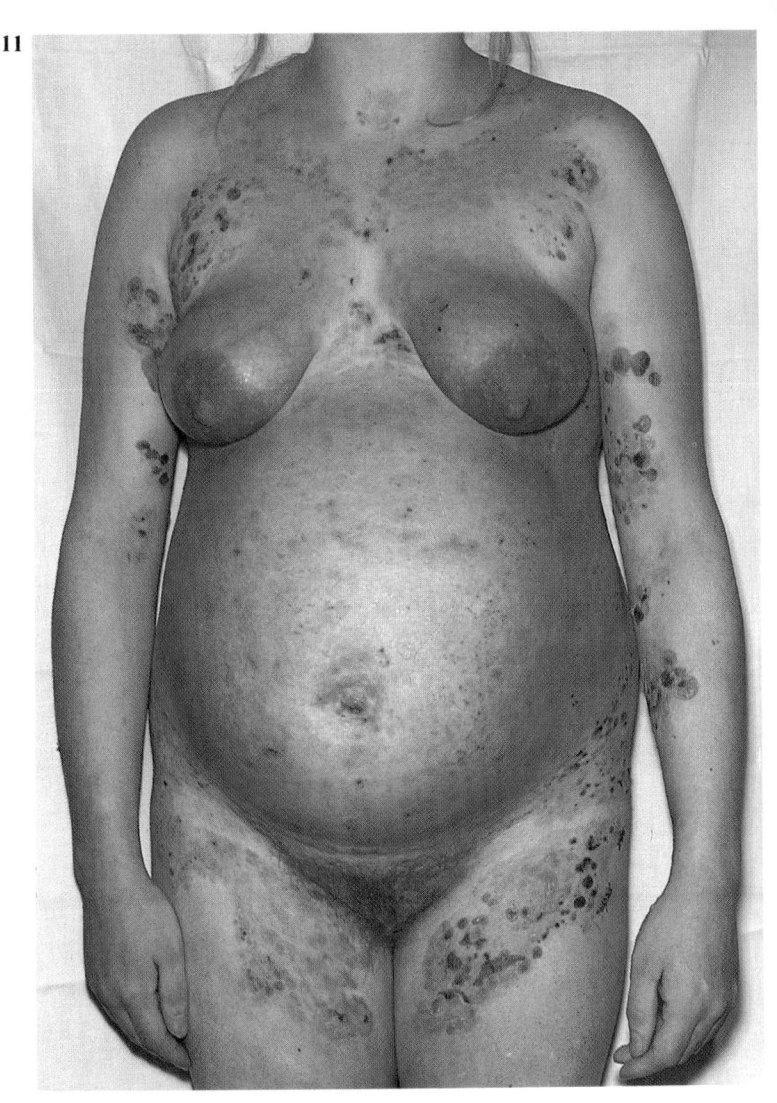

11 Intensely pruritic blistering eruption which the patient had suffered in a previous pregnancy and which recurred in the second trimester of this pregnancy.
(a) What is it?
(b) Which skin diseases are specifically associated with pregnancy.

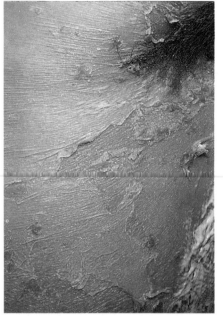

12

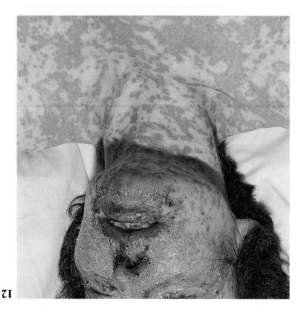

13

12, 13 Drug-induced eruption characterised by painful red patches with skin easily removed with gentle pressure.

(a) What is the most likely diagnosis?

(b) What are the known causes?

14

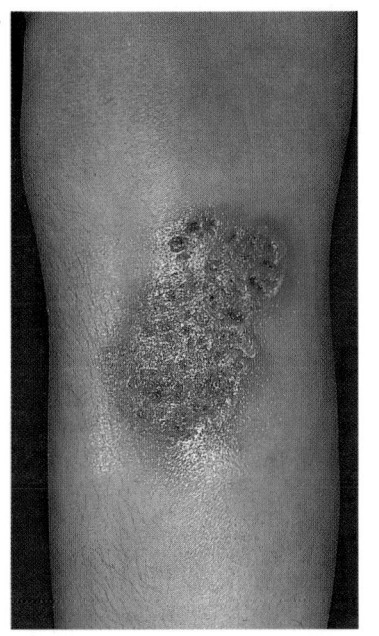

14 A young man with ulcerative colitis developed this rapidly enlarging ulcer below the knee. Purulent exudate from the ulcer failed to grow bacteria or fungi on culture.
(a) What is the diagnosis?
(b) With what diseases might it be associated?

15

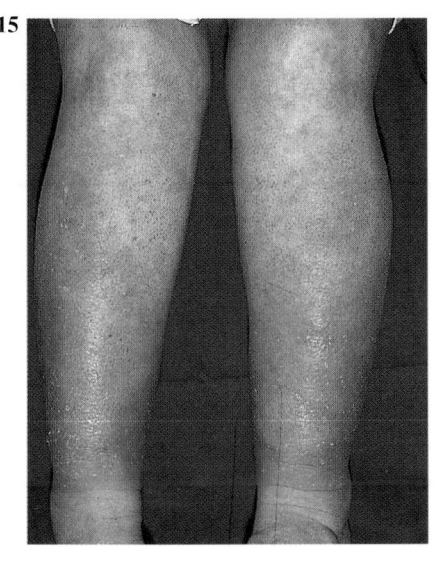

15 A 47-year-old woman complained of palpitations associated with weight loss. The shins showed diffuse plaques of non-pitting oedema.
(a) What is the probable diagnosis?
(b) What other signs would you look for?
(c) How would you treat the plaques over the shins?

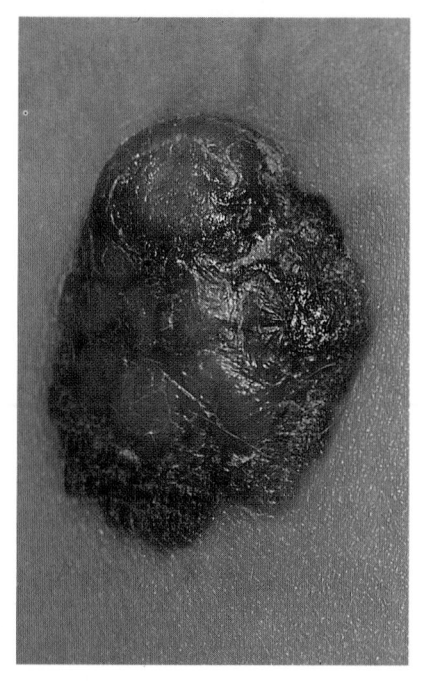

16, 17 Slowly growing pigmented lesion, 4 × 3 cm, on the thigh of a 32-year-old woman. The histology of the excised lesion is shown.
(a) What is it?
(b) Name other pigmented lesions which occasionally enter into the differential diagnosis.
(c) What are the features of the histology?

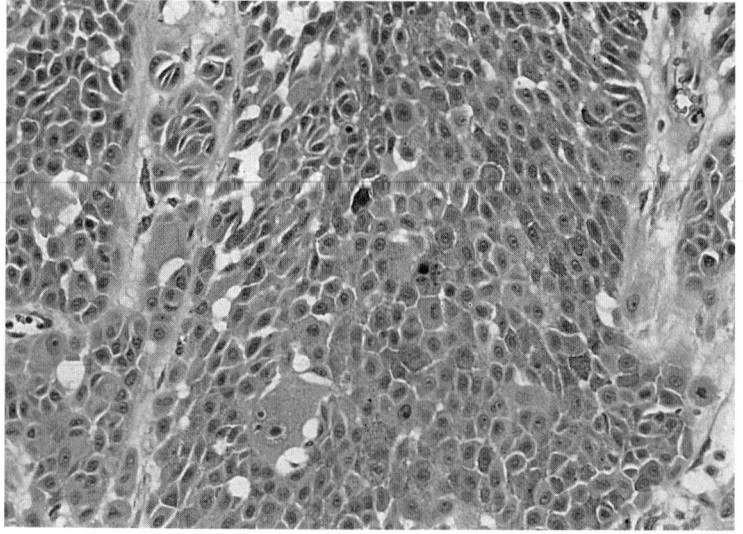

18 The hairdresser of this 27-year-old bricklayer noticed a collection of grey hairs over the occiput.
(a) What is the condition?
(b) With what may it be associated?
(c) Name three systemic diseases in which non-scarring alopecia may occur.

19 This man had dark-red telangiectatic papules, 1–2 mm diameter, symmetrically distributed on the posterior aspect of his thighs and elsewhere on the bathing trunk area. They form part of a rare hereditary disorder characterised also by renal failure, corneal opacities, vasomotor disturbances and hypertension.
(a) What is the disorder?
(b) What is the underlying cause?

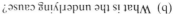

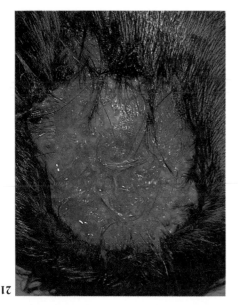

21 A scout grazed his scalp against the branch of a tree whilst on a nature trail. Three weeks later he presented with a grossly inflamed, alopecic plaque on the scalp.
(a) What is the diagnosis?
(b) How would you treat it?

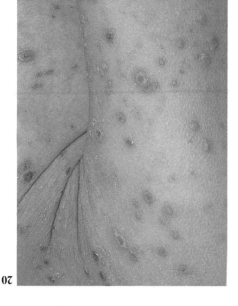

20 A child presented with pyrexia and a truncal eruption which consisted of papules, pustules and vesicles.
(a) What is the disease?
(b) What complications may occur?

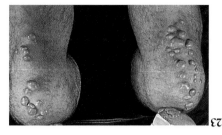

23 A milkman complained of intermittent claudication of recent onset.
Examination revealed orange-coloured nodules over the elbows and
knees.
(a) What is the condition?
(b) With what may it be associated?

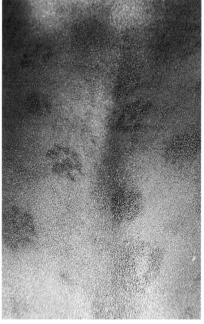

22 Pigmented patches since childhood on the back of a West African
patient. Extensive investigations revealed no evidence of systemic disease.
(a) How could the pigmentation have arisen?
(b) How would you treat it?

24 Pigmented lichenified pruritic dermatosis in a 7-year-old boy.
(a) What is it?
(b) In what other systemic diseases may a similar eruption occur?

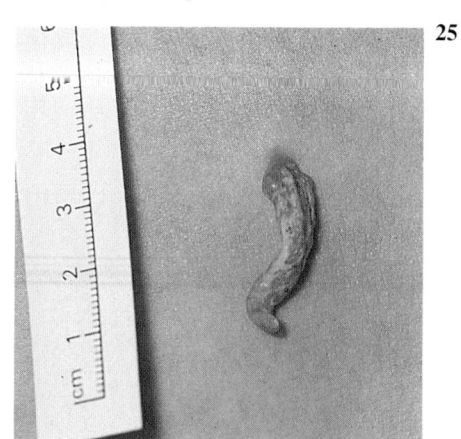

25 The horny outgrowth on the sternum of a 67-year-old man gradually increased in size.
(a) What is the common term for it?
(b) With what may it be associated?
(c) What complication may occur in longstanding lesions?

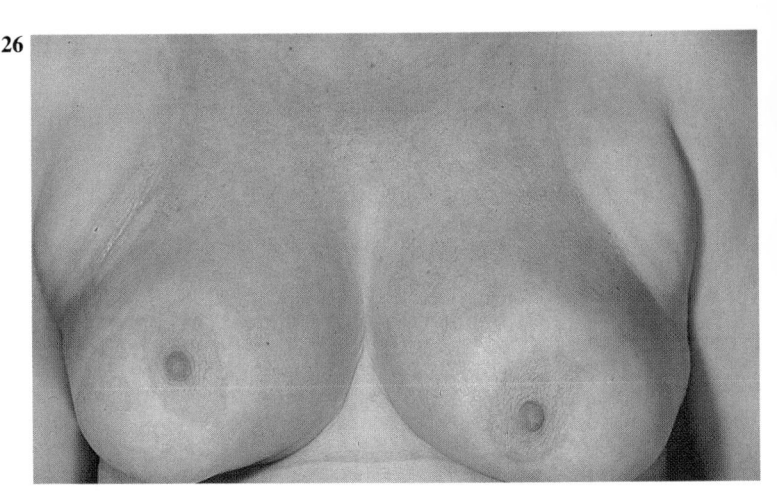

26 This lady presented with symmetrical, thickened, pigmented plaques over the breasts, abdomen and back. There was no associated lymphadenopathy.
(a) What is the diagnosis?
(b) How would you treat it?

27 Semicircular and arcuate lines over the thumbnails of an anxious shopkeeper.
(a) What is the cause?
(b) What should it be differentiated from?

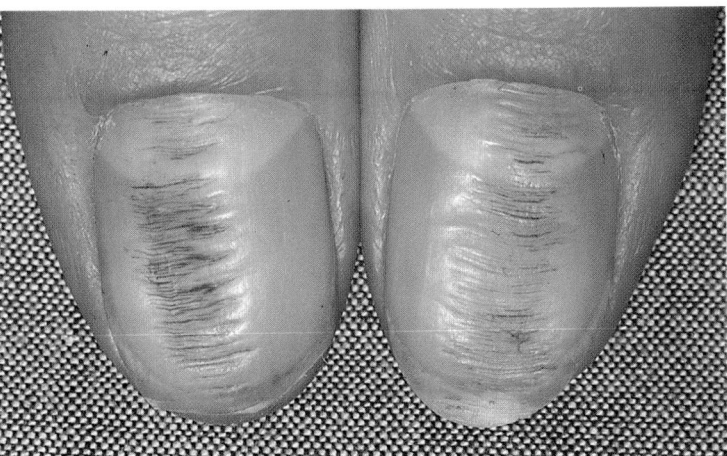

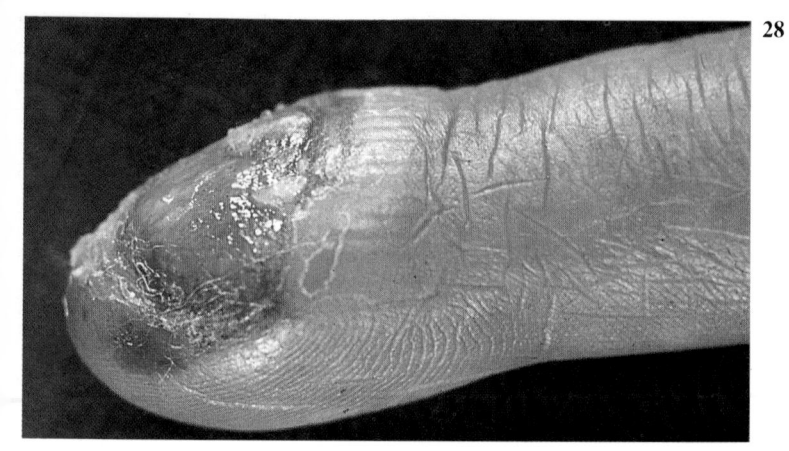

28 A carpenter injured his index finger several months previously. He next presented with a non-healing wound.
(a) What physical signs indicate that this is not a simple wound?
(b) What is the likely diagnosis?

29 (a) What treatment has caused this reaction?
(b) What other complications may occur from this treatment?

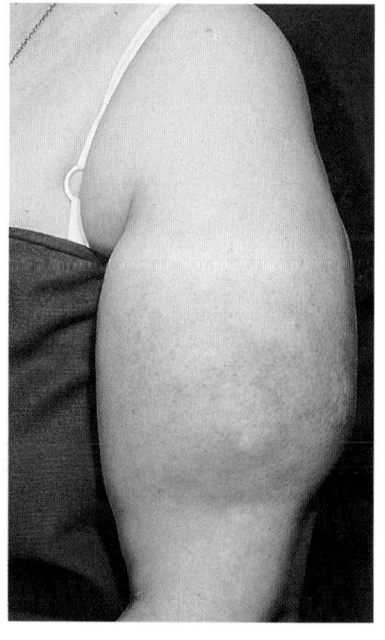

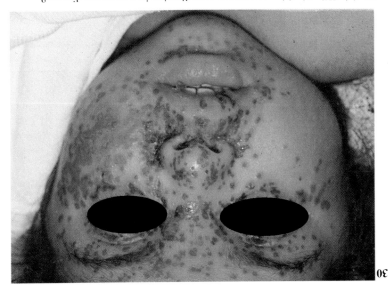

30 (a) What is this uncommon complication in a common disease?
(b) What is the cause?
(c) What complications might ensue from the disease?

31 Warts appeared in a middle-aged lady's axillae, and velvety thickening and hyperpigmentation were noted over the neck, axillae and groins.

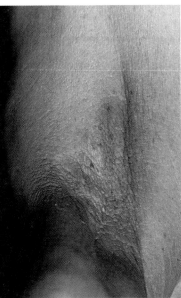

(a) What is this condition?
(b) What other signs would you look for?
(c) What other conditions may be associated?

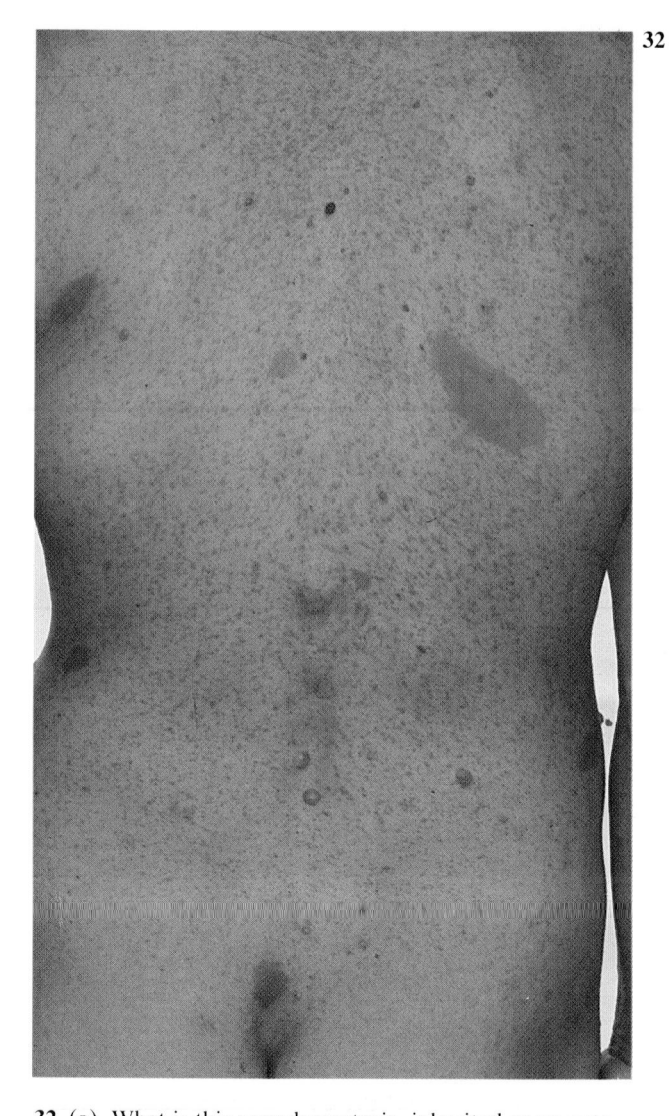

32 (a) What is this genodermatosis, inherited as an auto-somal dominant gene?
(b) Describe significant features of the disease.

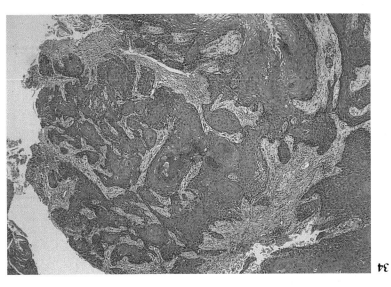

34

33, 34 A rapidly growing tumour and its histology (34) in a 78-year-old sailor.
(a) What is the diagnosis?
(b) Name three other tumours which may affect the ear.

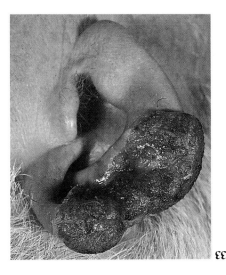

33

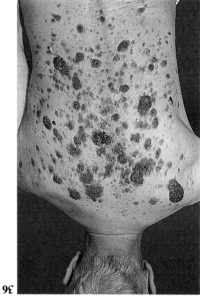

35 (a) What is this important physical sign?
(b) What is its significance?

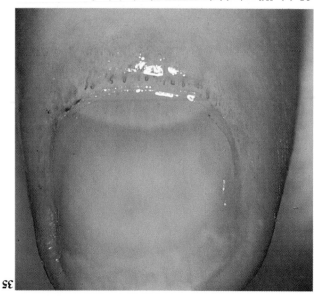

36 (a) What are these pigmented tumours in a 67-
year-old ex-miner?
(b) What is their significance?

37

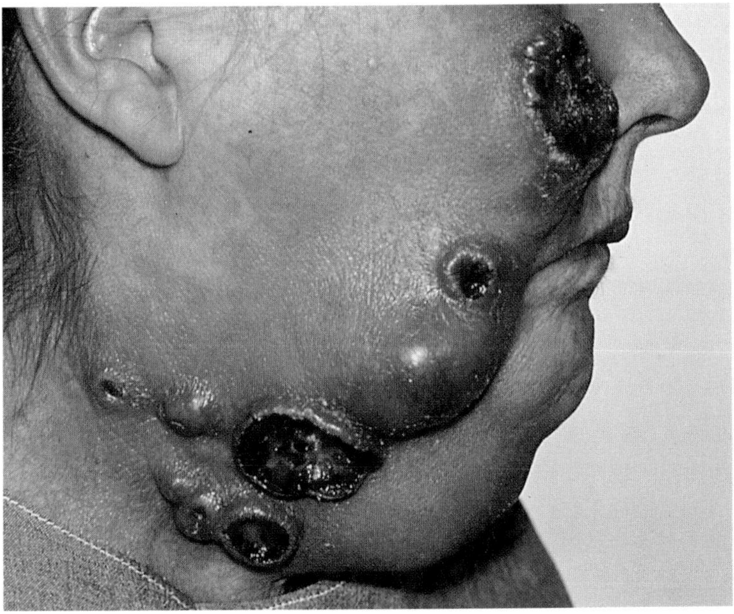

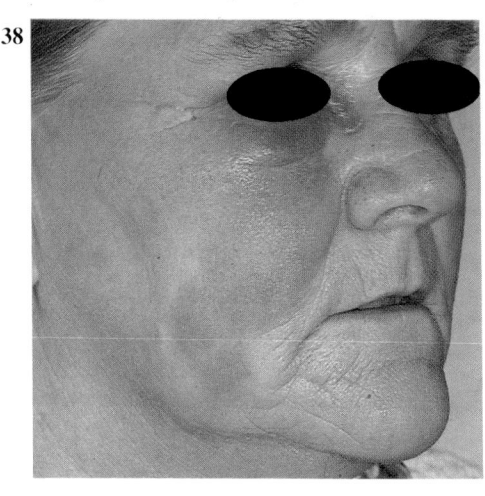

37 A late complication of an increasingly common cutaneous neoplasm.
(a) What is it?
(b) What aetiological factors are thought to be relevant in the development of the primary lesion?

38 (a) What is the cause of the facial eruption in this 'latent' diabetic?
(b) What factors increase susceptibility to it?

39 A man presented with acute abdominal pain and these auricular 'tumours'.
(a) What are they?
(b) How may the abdominal pain be related?

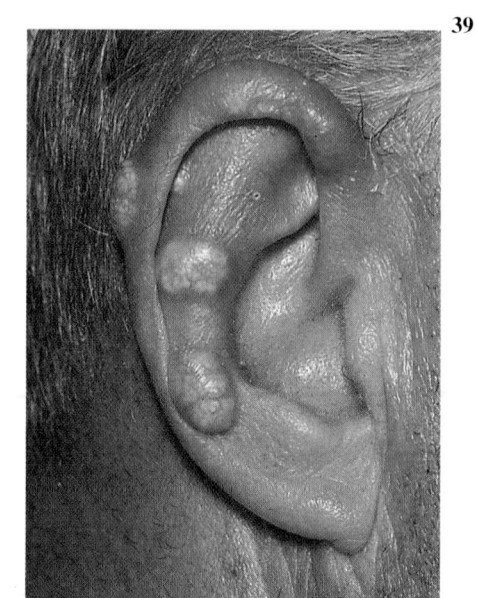

40 A rapidly growing tumour on a 42-year-old man's cheek.
(a) What is the tumour?
(b) What must it be distinguished from?

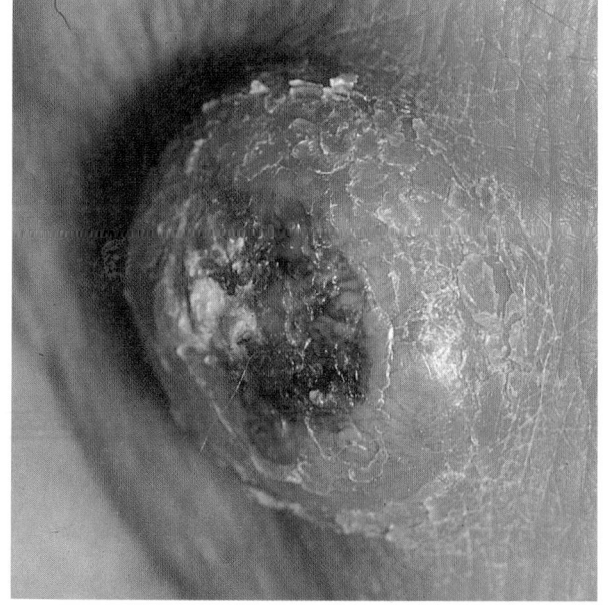

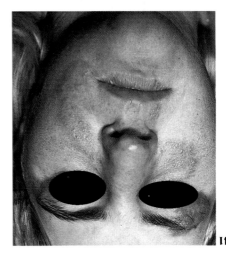

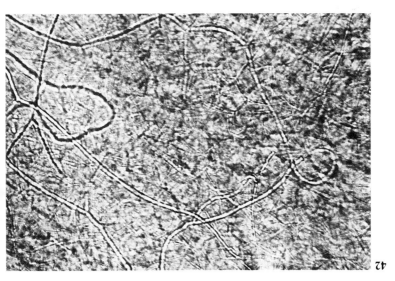

41, 42 An asymmetrical facial eruption made worse with topical steroids.
Microscopy of skin scrapings (42) revealed the reason.
(a) What is the eruption?
(b) What does microscopy show?

43 This young man complained of burning of the skin a few minutes after exposure to sunlight. The facial skin showed scars and premature wrinkling.
(a) What disease do you suspect?
(b) How would you confirm the diagnosis?

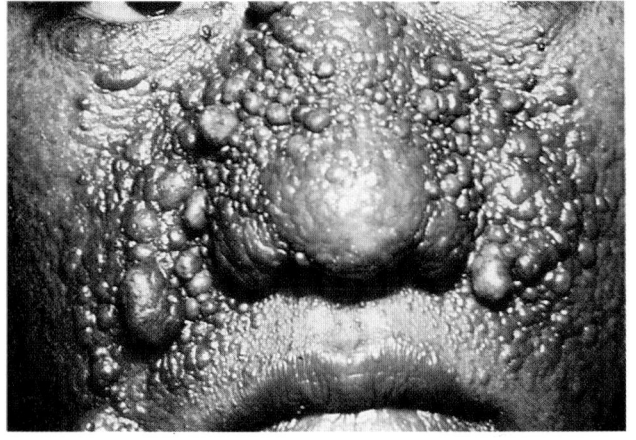

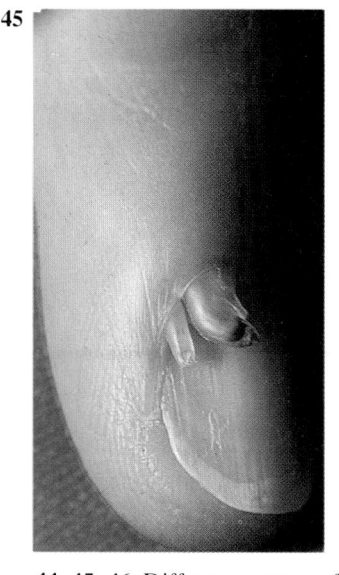 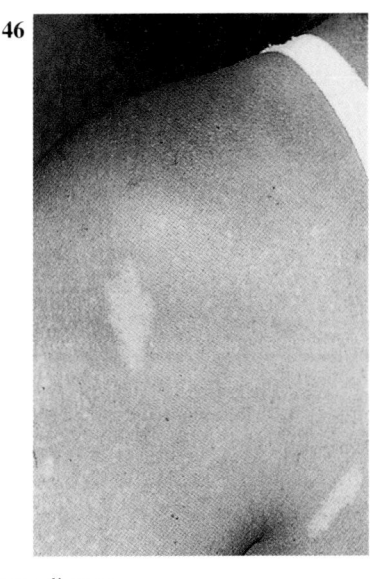

44, 45, 46 Different aspects of the same disease.
(a) What is the disease?
(b) Name other cutaneous features of the condition.

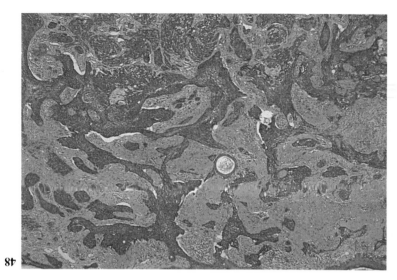

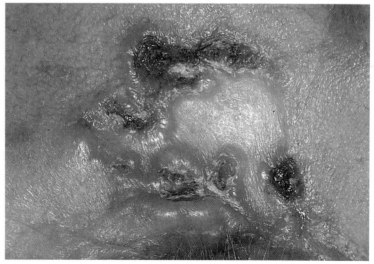

47, 48 Infiltrating tumour over the cheek with histology of the raised margin.

(a) What is it?
(b) What may give rise to it?
(c) What does the histology show?

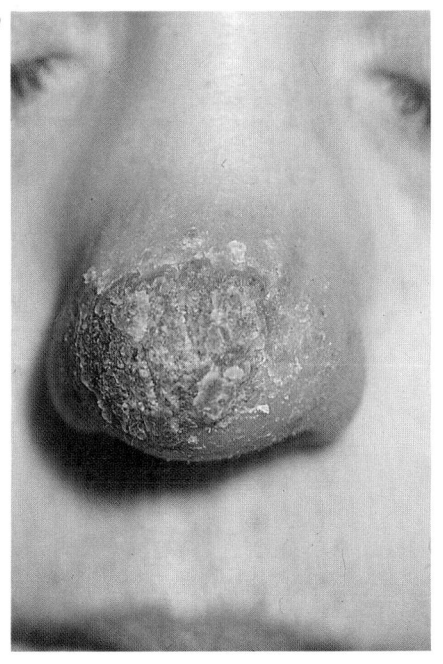

49 The cutaneous sequel of a tropical disease particularly common around the Mediterranean coast.
(a) What is it?
(b) How may it be acquired?

50 An infantile form of what is usually a post-pubertal disorder.
(a) What is the condition?
(b) What systemic disease should you exclude?

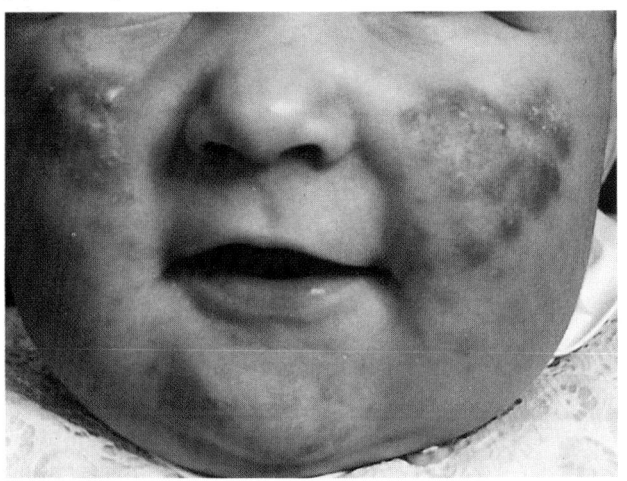

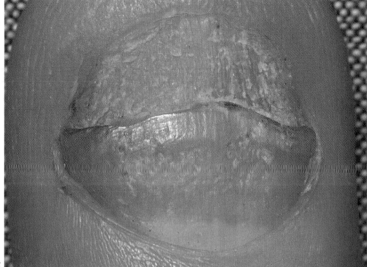

52

51 Atrophic scars on the knee of a boy who complained of easy bruising.
(a) What is it?
(b) Name some other features of the disease?

52 An artefactual alteration of a finger-nail showing features associated with a common dermatosis.
(a) What is the dermatosis?
(b) What nail changes occur?

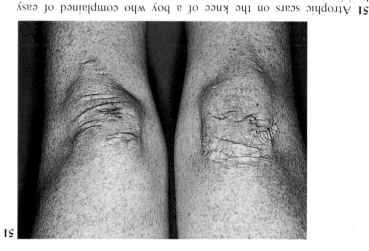

51

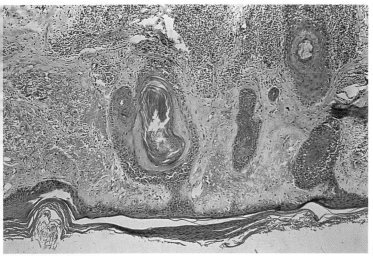

54

53 (a) What is this circumoral dermatosis?
(b) What may cause it?

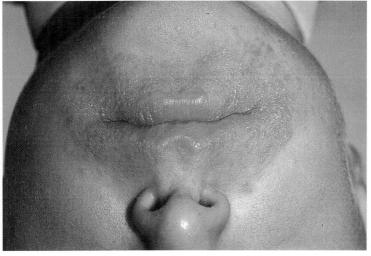

53

54, 55 A lady had a persistent, red, scaly eruption with scars on her face; the histology of a skin biopsy is shown.
(a) What is the diagnosis?
(b) How can the diagnosis be confirmed?
(c) What is the prognosis?
(d) What features appear in the skin biopsy?

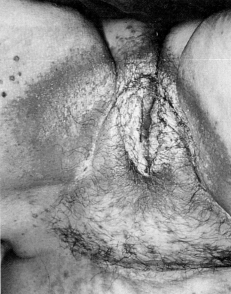

57 Intensely pruritic perineal eruption associated with a profuse vaginal discharge.
(a) What is it?
(b) Name some predisposing factors.

57

56 A 'positive' skin test in a patient with von Willebrand's disease.
(a) What is the test?
(b) How would you perform it?
(c) What is its significance?

56

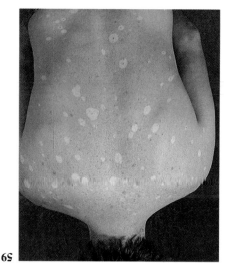

59 A bricklayer fond of the sun noticed an increasing number of white patches over his chest and back. Antifungal therapy was un-helpful.

(a) What is the diagnosis?
(b) With what may it be associated?

58 A man with recurrent chest infections complained that for several months his nails had virtually ceased to grow. Examination revealed discoloured nails but fungal culture was negative.

(a) What is the condition?
(b) With what may it be associated?
(c) Name one other possible cause for the nail colour.

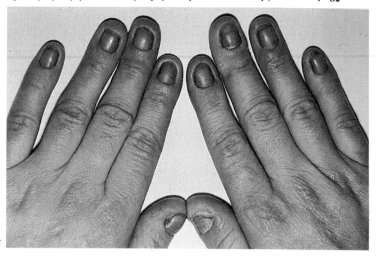

60 Buccal mucosal changes associated with a papular, purplish eruption over the wrists and forearms.
(a) What is the mucosal eruption?
(b) Name the conditions which may present as white lesions in the mouth.

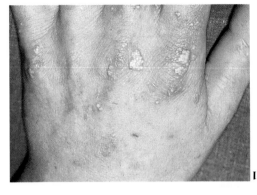

61 An alcoholic with scarring and multiple milia formation over the dorsum of the hands.
(a) What is the disease?
(b) Which other systemic disorder is frequently associated?

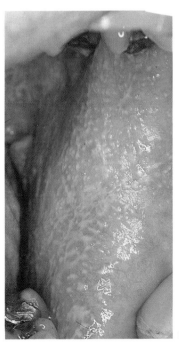

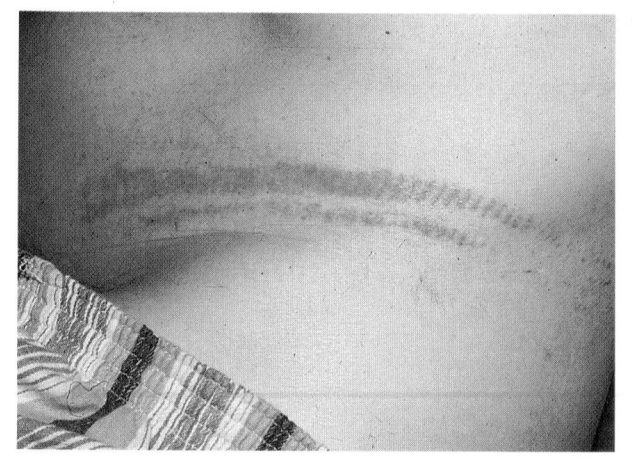

66 An inpatient blamed a plaster dressing for this eruption on his abdomen.
(a) What was the real cause?
(b) How would you prove it?

67 The patient was referred as 'a collection of warts unresponsive to conventional therapy'.
(a) What is the true diagnosis?
(b) What is the natural history of the condition?

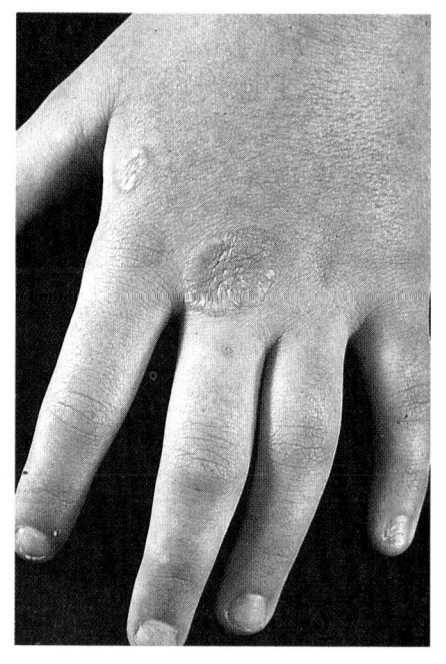

68

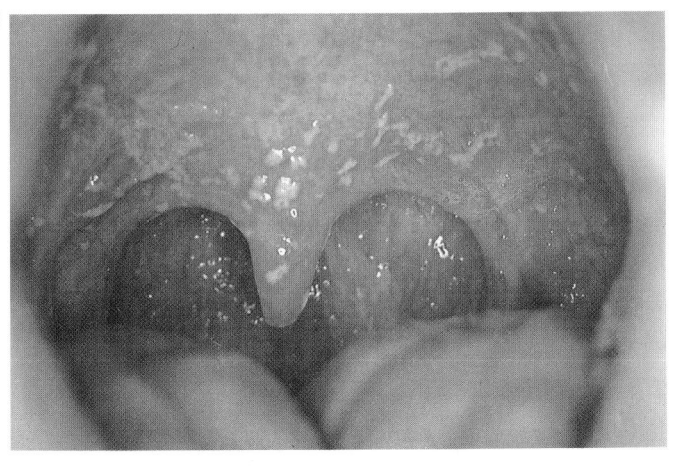

69

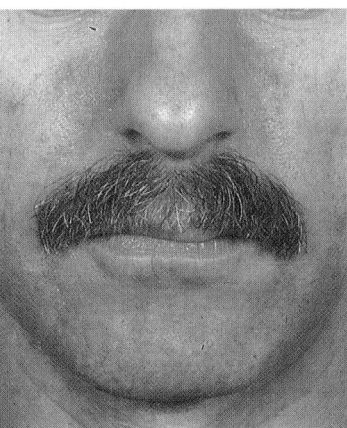

68, 69, 70 This young man gave a short history of a sore throat, a facial eruption and superficial painless, purpuric nodules on his neck and elsewhere. The platelet count was normal.
(a) What are the lesions?
(b) With which serious disorder may they be associated?

(c) How would a social history help in the diagnosis?
(d) Name other cutaneous manifestations of this disease.

71 Haemorrhagic bulla in the morning is a 'shepherd's warning'!
(a) What is it?
(b) How would you treat it?

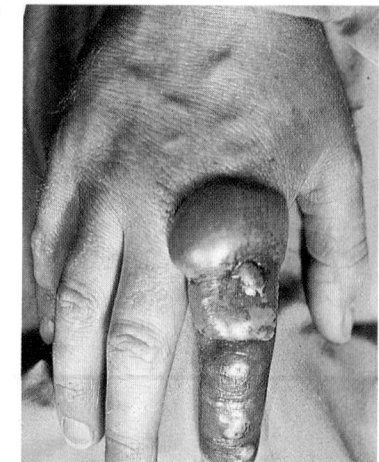

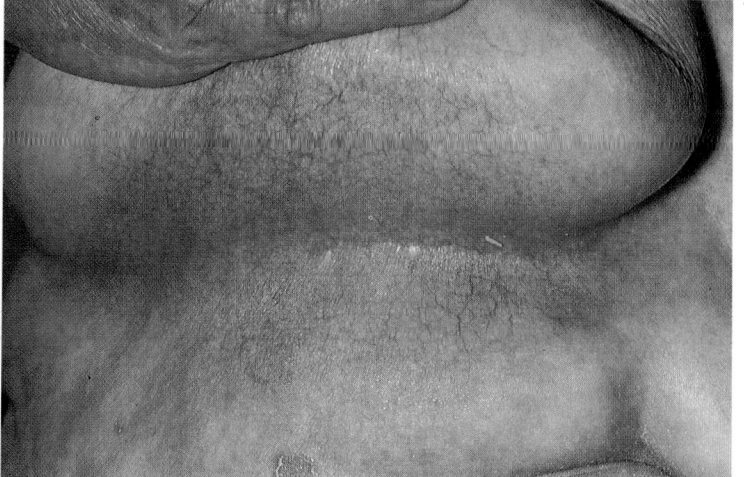

72 A not uncommon side effect from the prolonged use of a topical medication
(a) What is it?
(b) What are other recognised side effects?

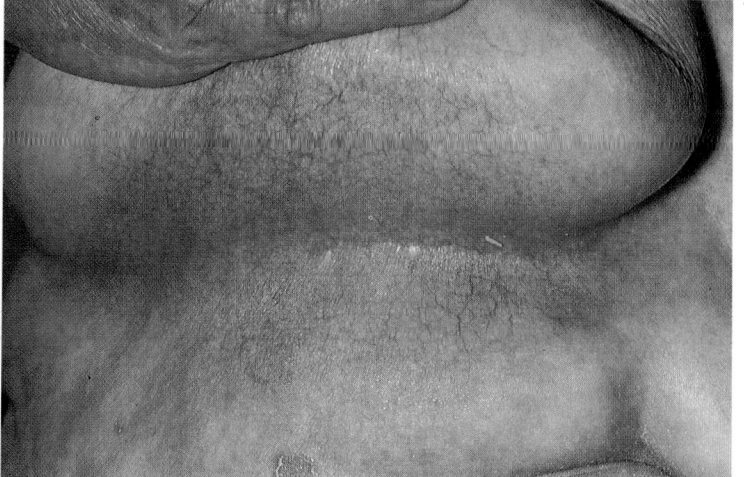

73

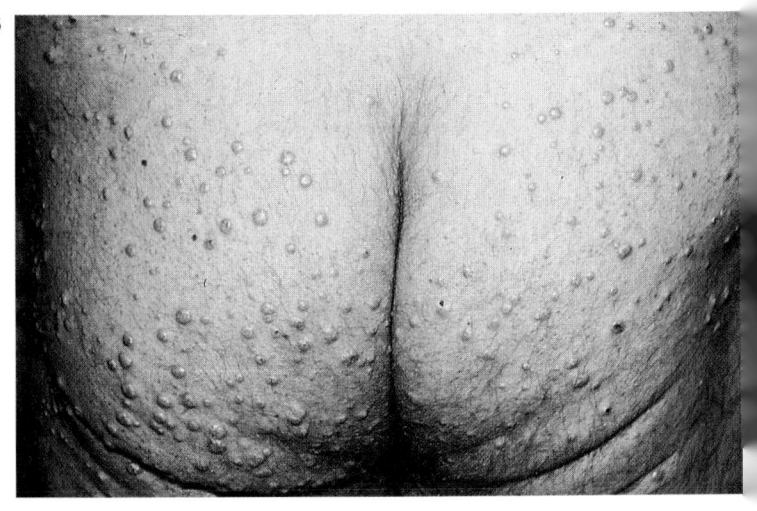

73 An uncontrolled diabetic developed this profuse eruption.
(a) What are the lesions?
(b) What other clinical varieties are described?

74 The result of a common world-wide infection.
(a) What physical signs are apparent?
(b) What is the cause?

74

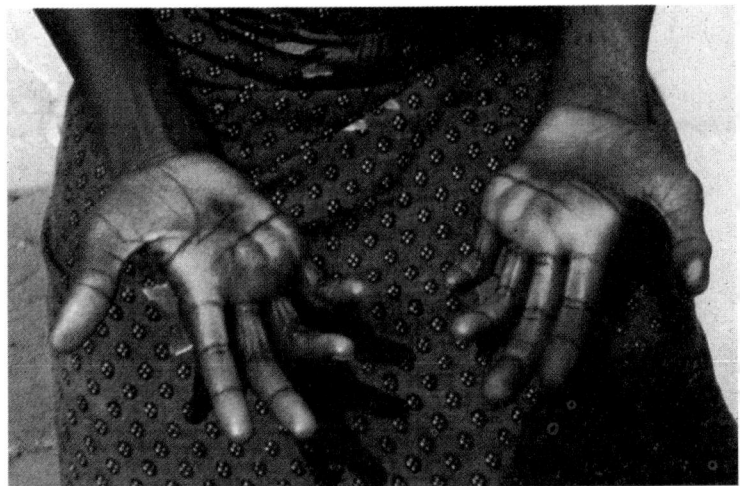

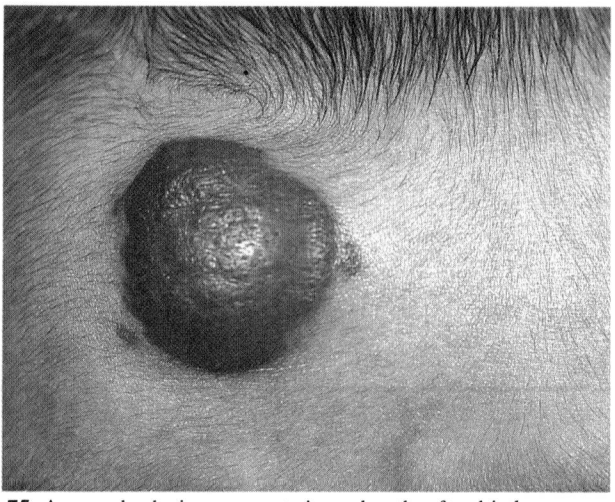

75 A vascular lesion present since shortly after birth.
(a) What is it?
(b) What treatment would you recommend?

76 A 32-year-old lady complained of a hoarse voice. Examination revealed a profuse nodular eruption over the face, chest and buttocks. A chest X-ray provided confirmatory evidence.
(a) What is the disease likely to be?
(b) To what was the hoarseness due?
(c) What did the chest X-ray show?

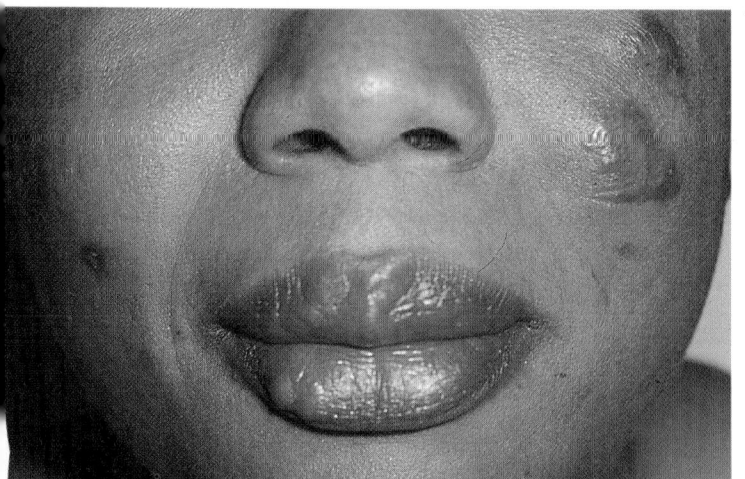

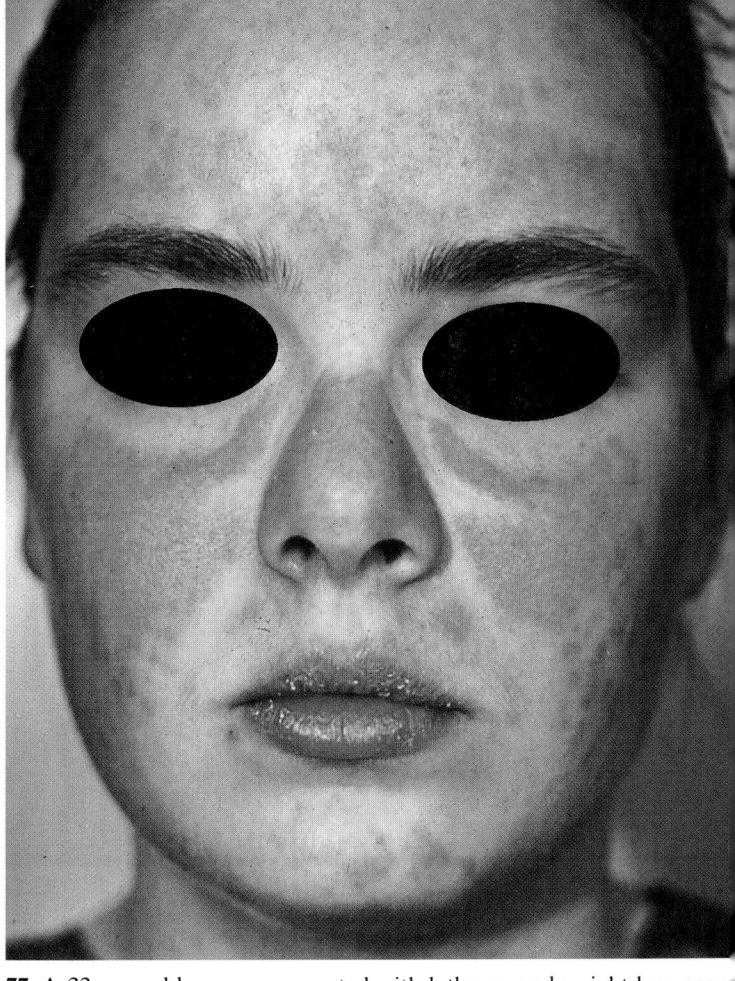

77 A 22-year-old woman presented with lethargy and weight loss occurring over two months. General examination was unhelpful and a Monospot test was negative. On holiday after a couple of days' exposure to sunlight she developed this facial eruption.
(a) What is the probable diagnosis?
(b) Which other cutaneous signs can occur in the disease.
(c) List some complications of the systemic disorder.

78 An East African lady presented with shortness of breath, weight loss, easy fatigability and a superficially ulcerated scaly lesion over the face. General examination of the skin otherwise normal. A chest X-ray suggested the cause for the dyspnoea.

(a) What was the cause of the skin lesion?

(b) What clinical varieties occur?

(c) What complications occur in longstanding disease?

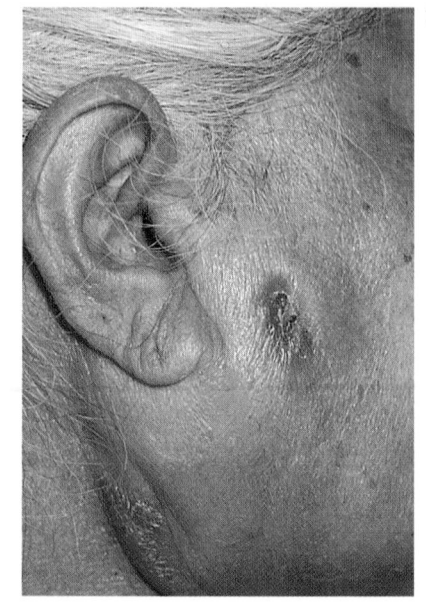

79 A 37-year-old librarian presented with a slowly growing red nodule behind her left ear. First noticed six months previously, it occasionally became sore.

(a) What physical sign helps in diagnosis?

(b) What is the usual cause?

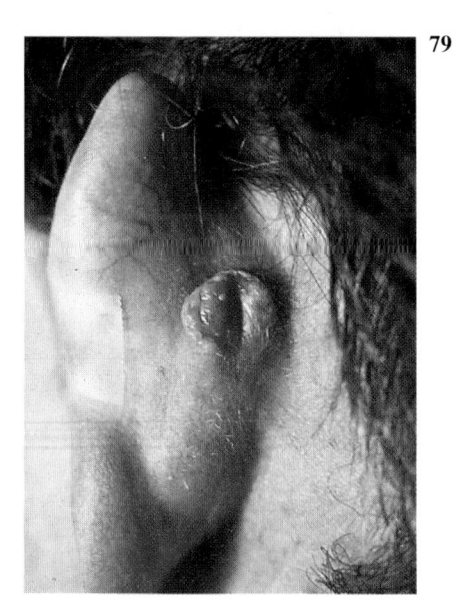

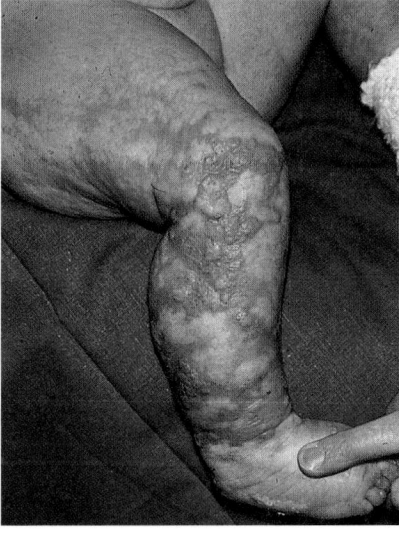

80 This 42-year-old West African patient presented with an erythematous mildly scaly plaque over the right side of the face. The left side of the face and the rest of the skin appeared normal. The neck revealed an enlarged nerve.
(a) What is the diagnosis?
(b) What other physical signs may be present?
(c) Which other nerves should be examined?

81 Blisters developed soon after birth in this baby girl. The bullae became recurrent and blister fluid failed to show bacteria or virus on culture. It was observed that the blisters were often distributed in a linear fashion. The infant subsequently formed pigmented patches.
(a) What is this hereditary disorder?
(b) What other systems, apart from the skin, may be involved?

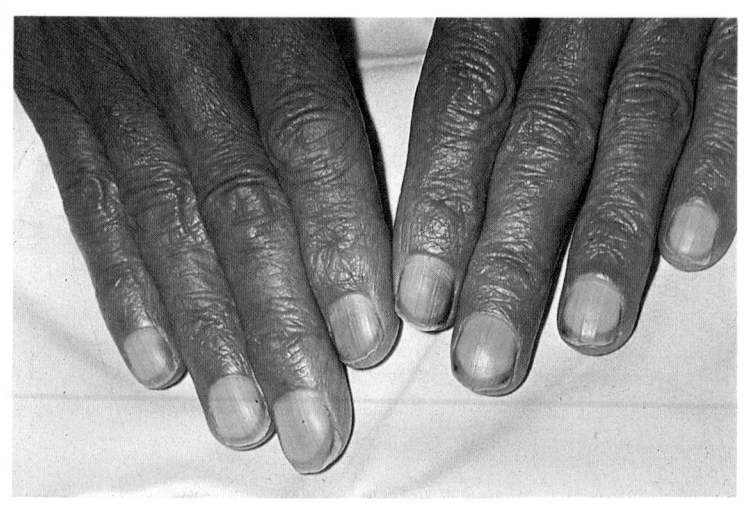

82 A 37-year-old brewery worker presented with weakness and anorexia. He had a painless hepatomegaly.
(a) What are the nails associated with?
(b) Name other nail changes associated with systemic disease.

83 This woman was admitted with right-sided chest pain. General examination, chest X-ray and ECG showed no abnormality. Five days later, a vesicular eruption developed over the right breast which, by the 7th day became florid and associated with this widespread eruption.
(a) What is the condition?
(b) What precautions are advisable?
(c) What trigger factors are recognised?

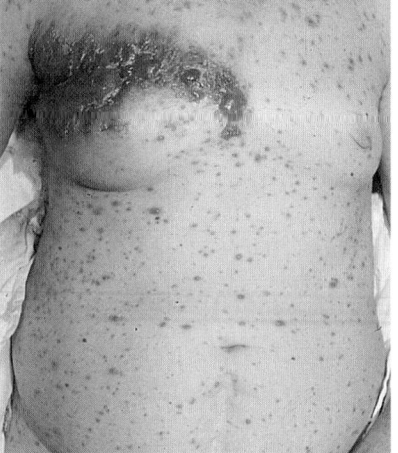

84

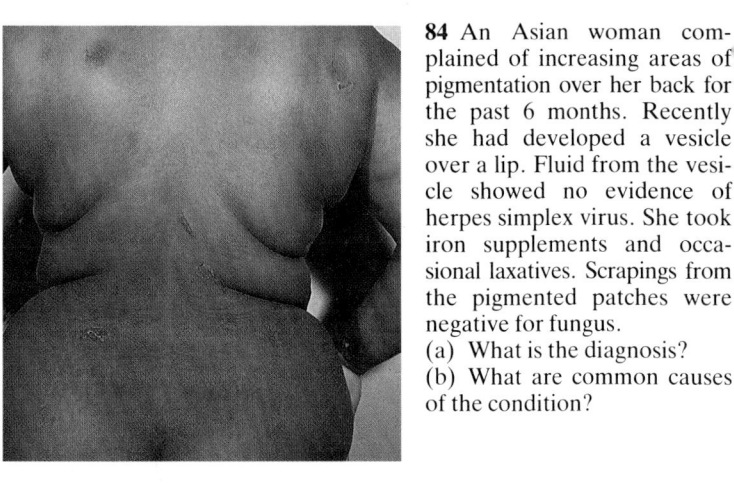

84 An Asian woman complained of increasing areas of pigmentation over her back for the past 6 months. Recently she had developed a vesicle over a lip. Fluid from the vesicle showed no evidence of herpes simplex virus. She took iron supplements and occasional laxatives. Scrapings from the pigmented patches were negative for fungus.
(a) What is the diagnosis?
(b) What are common causes of the condition?

85 A young man presented with scarring and papulopustules over his back. He first developed lesions over his face, chest and back 5 years previously, when he had been prescribed antibiotics with good results. He had not continued with therapy as recommended.
(a) What was his initial condition?
(b) Name some aetiological factors.
(c) Is there an inherited pre-disposition to the condition?

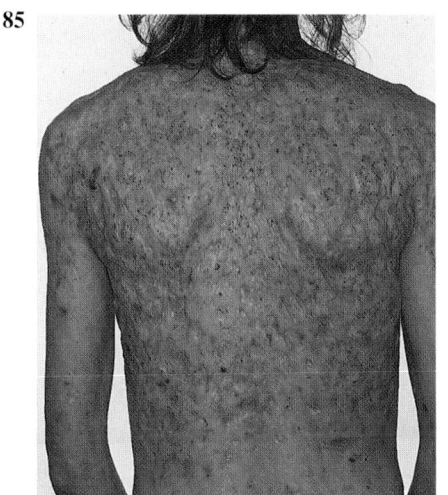

85

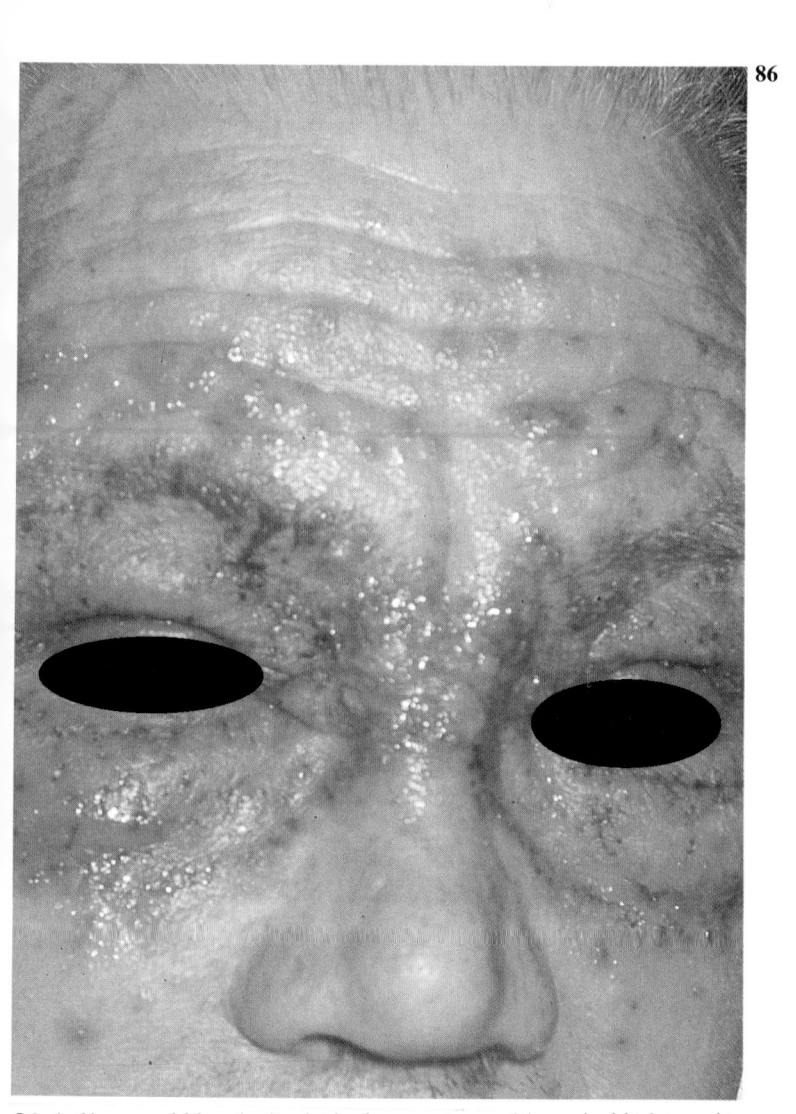

86 A 61-year-old horticulturist had an acute pruritic periorbital eruption. He improved with topical steroids but the eruption reappeared on his return to work.
(a) What is the probable diagnosis?
(b) What causes should you consider?
(c) How would you confirm the cause?

87

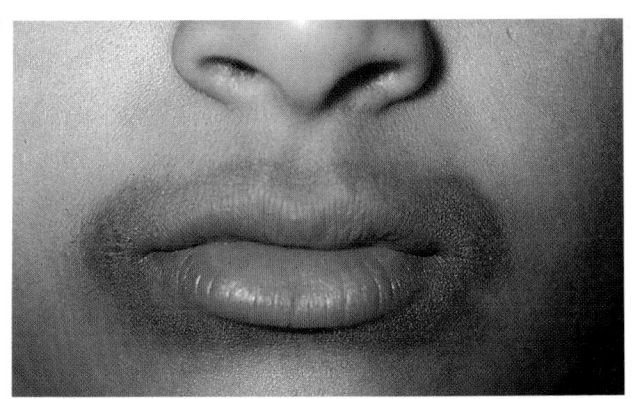

87 A boy presented with a circumoral scaly eruption. With no history of skin disease and of good general health, his parents described him as being of a nervous disposition.
(a) What is the condition?
(b) What would you include in the differential diagnosis?

88

88 An erythematous scaly eruption over the face associated with greasy scales over the scalp.
(a) What is the condition?
(b) Where else should you look for a rash?
(c) What conditions need to be excluded?

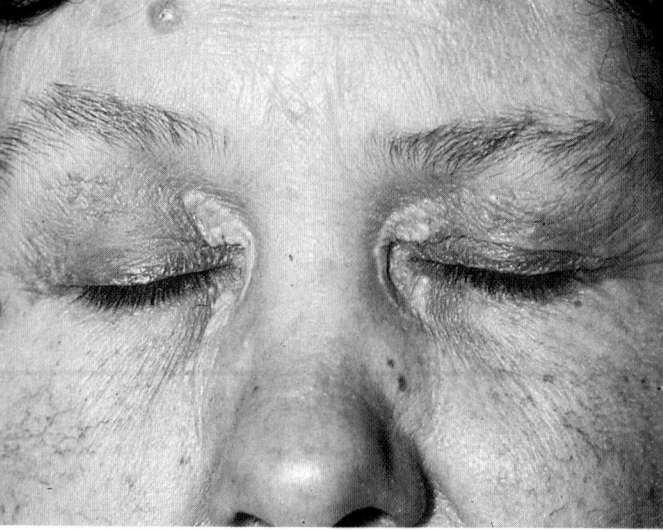

89 (a) What are these asymptomatic yellowish plaques over the inner canthi?
(b) Name three recognised causes.
(c) How may the lesions be treated?

90 The skin of the right side of the neck shows telangiectasia as a result of overdosage of a therapeutic measure.
(a) What is the cutaneous reaction?
(b) What other complications may ensue?

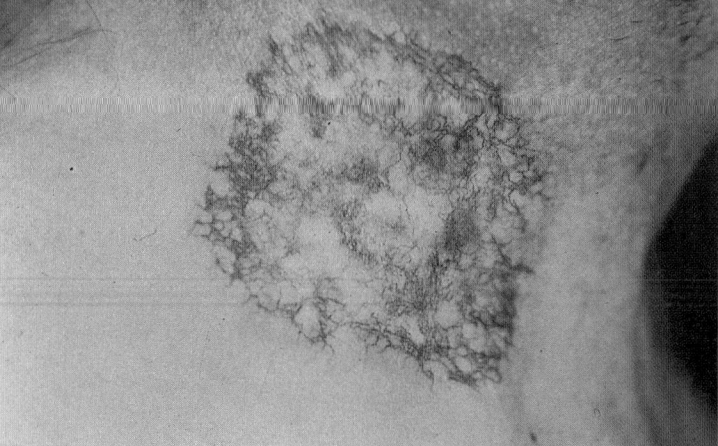

91

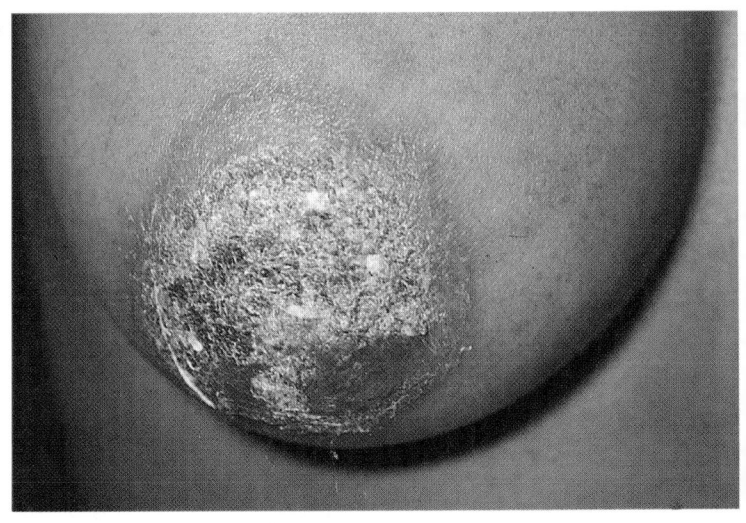

91, 92 The same breast before and after treatment of a longstanding eruption.
(a) What is the condition most likely to be?
(b) What features suggest that it is not a malignant process?

92

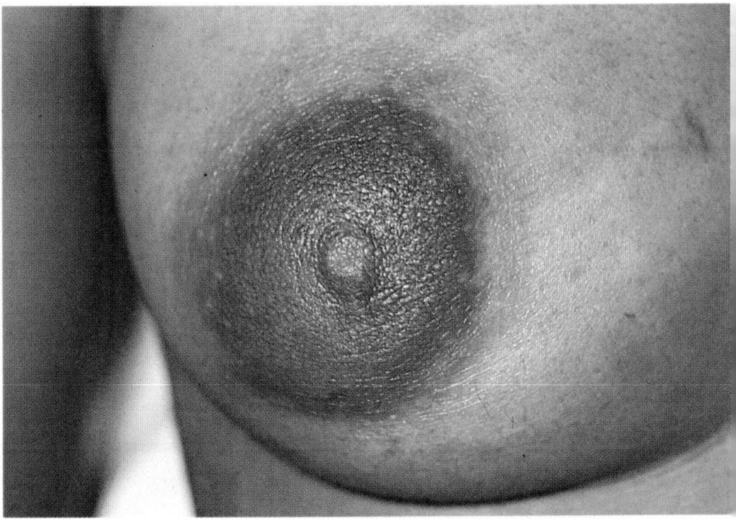

93 Firm dome-shaped lesions behind the ear in a patient with acne vulgaris.
(a) What are they?
(b) What complication of similar lesions in sternal skin could give a confusing image on chest X-ray.

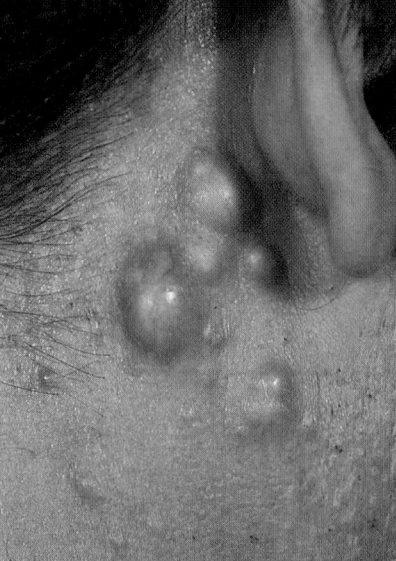

93

94 Common warty lesions over the face of an Afro-Caribbean woman.
(a) What are they?
(b) What is their significance?

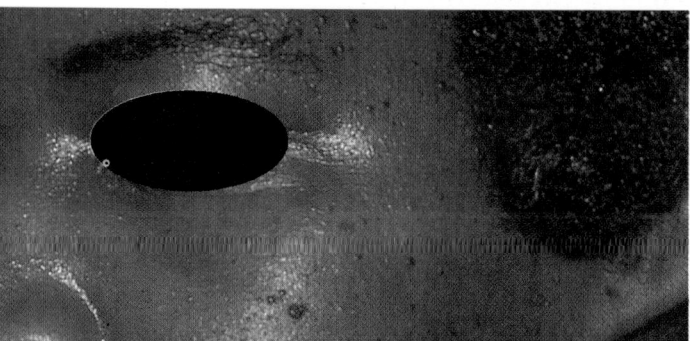

94

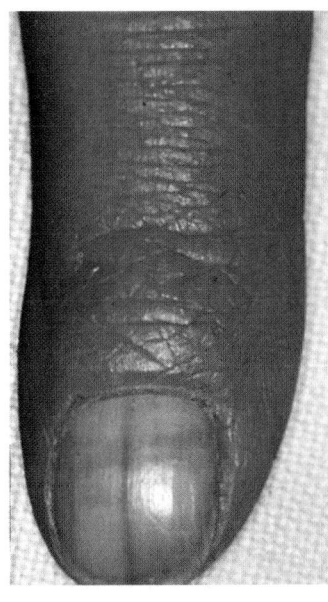

95 A linear band of pigment in a nail. This patient developed similar bands in other finger-nails.
(a) What is the condition?
(b) What complication may occur?

96 A young woman presented with an acute abdomen and gave a two-year history of colicky abdominal pain, accompanied by borborygmi. At first the attacks were mild but in recent weeks had become severe and prolonged. There was epigastric tenderness and a mass extending from the epigastrium to the left hypochondrium. The buccal mucosa showed pigmentation and there were lesions around the mouth.
(a) What is the diagnosis?
(b) Name an important though uncommon complication?

96

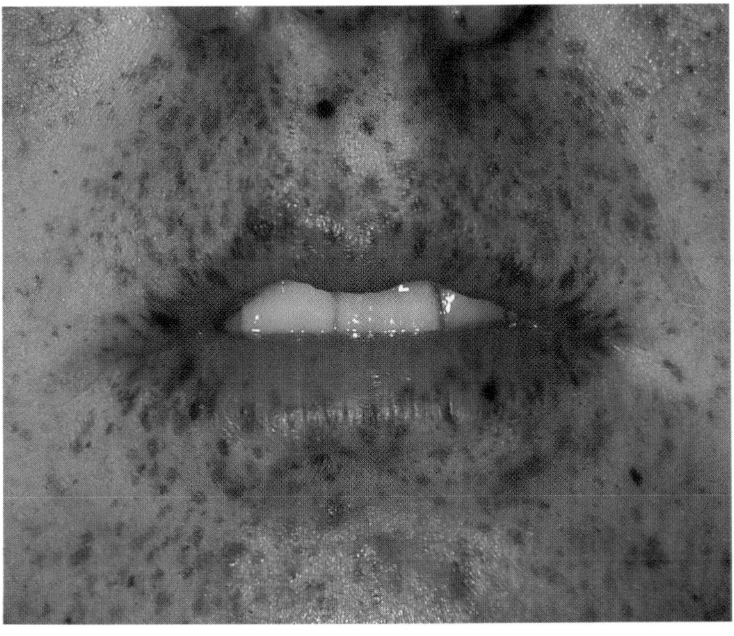

![Image 96]

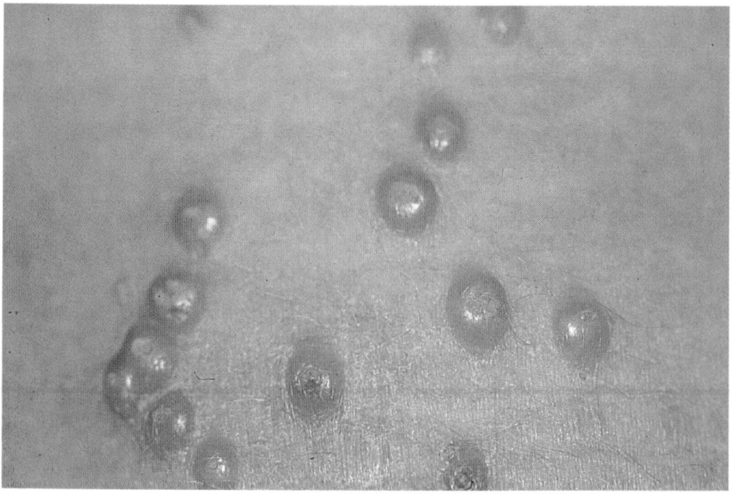

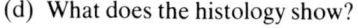

97, 98 These pale papules (2 mm in diameter) arose on the front of the neck of a 5-year-old boy and had been present for about 2 months. The clinical appearance is characteristic, as is the histology (**98**, obtained from an adult patient with similar lesions).

(a) What are they?
(b) What causes them?
(c) What patients are at particular risk from developing them?
(d) What does the histology show?

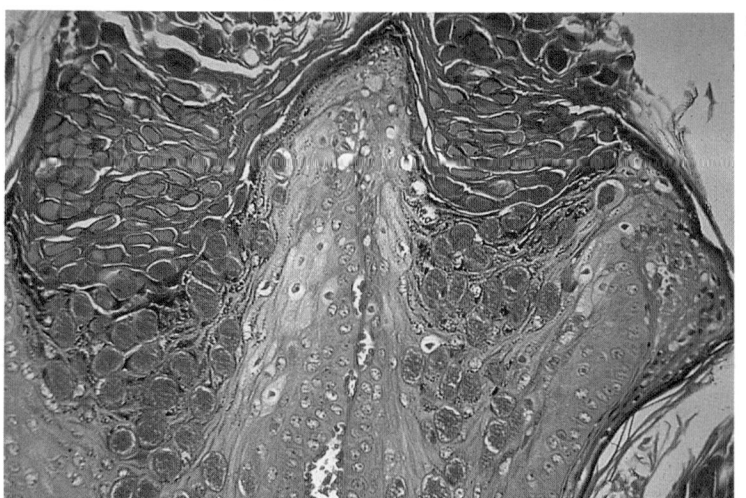

99

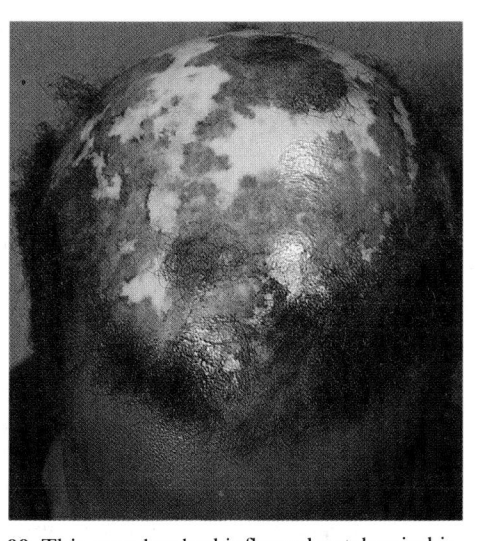

99 This man has had inflamed patches in his scalp for many years and now has permanent hair loss with pigmentary changes.
(a) What is the likely diagnosis?
(b) What other conditions can result in scarring alopecia?

100

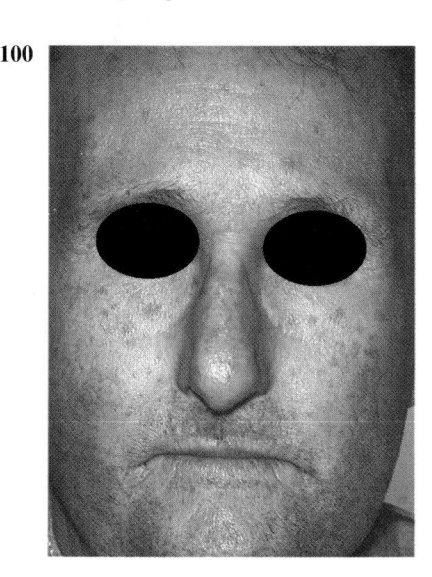

100 A 47-year-old man suffered shortness of breath on mild exertion; chest X-ray showed changes consistent with pulmonary fibrosis. He had blanching of the fingers, particularly on exposure to cold. The facies suggested the diagnosis.
(a) What is the diagnosis?
(b) What other physical signs might be found?

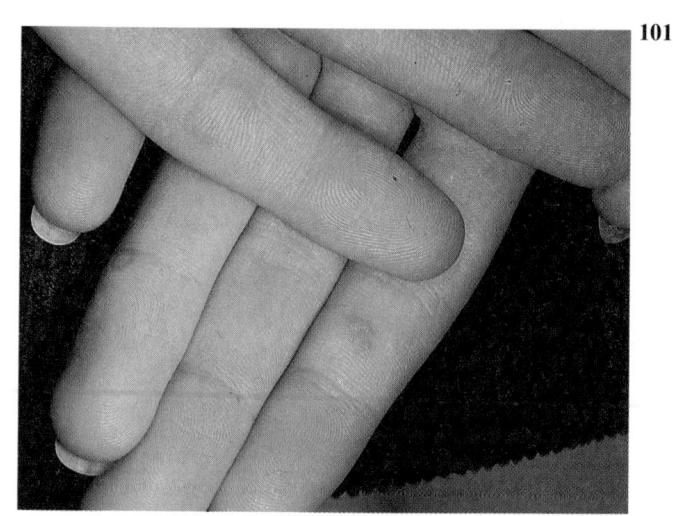

101 This girl's vesicles developed about a week after being in contact with a child who had similar lesions.
(a) What is the disorder?
(b) Where else would you look for lesions?
(c) What is the usual causative organism?
(d) How would you confirm the diagnosis?

102 (a) What is the name given to this shape of ear?
(b) What does it tell you about his past life?
(c) By what mechanism is the deformity produced?

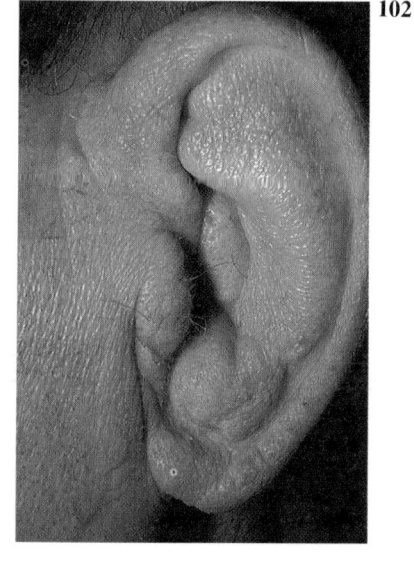

103

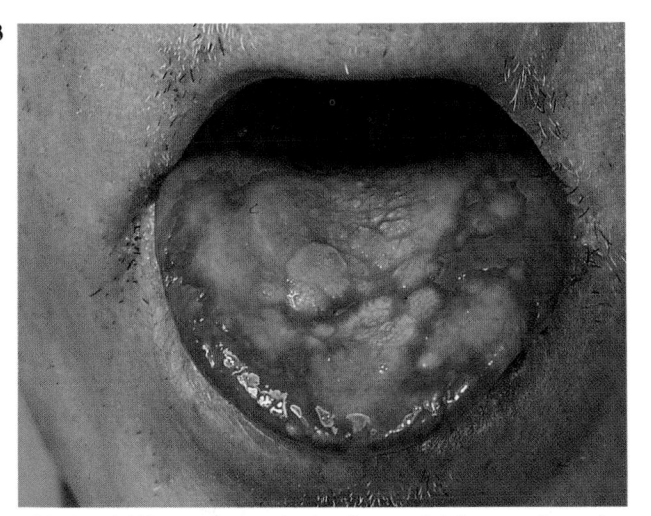

103 A middle-aged man had a 3-month history of an ulcerated tongue and a very itchy eruption on his wrists and ankles.
(a) What is this likely to be?
(b) What other conditions cause persistent or recurrent mouth ulceration?

104 A girl has developed a smooth round bald patch on the scalp.
(a) What is this most likely to be?
(b) What is the prognosis?
(c) Name some other causes of patchy hair loss in a child?

104

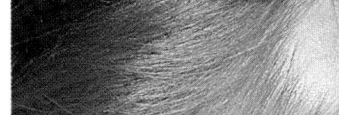

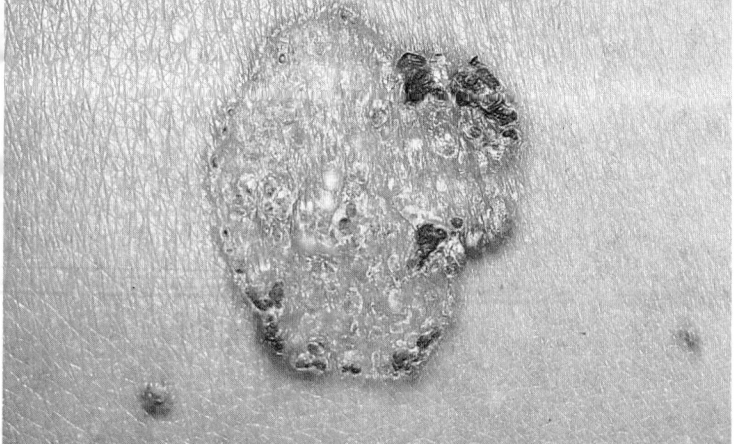

105 The patient has excoriated lichenified dermatitis in the knee flexures.
(a) This appearance, particularly in children, is virtually pathognomonic of which type of dermatitis?
(b) Where else would you look for skin lesions of similar type?
(c) What other medical disorders tend to be associated more frequently in these patients and their families?

106 A well demarcated scaly patch, 15mm across, and with a raised margin was situated on the back of a middle-aged man.
(a) What is it?
(b) How will a detailed history help to explain its presence?
(c) How can it be treated?
(d) From what should it be differentiated?

107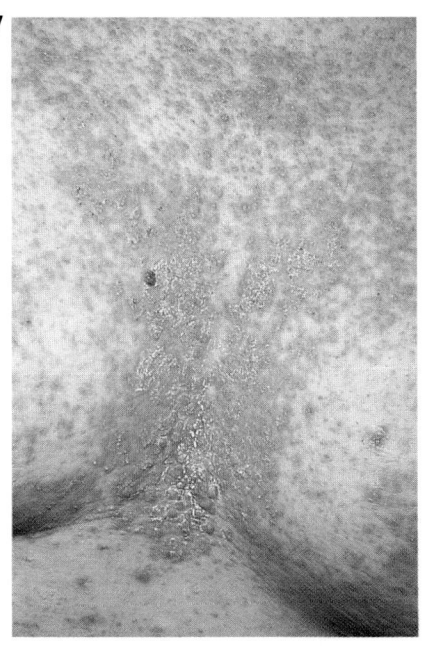

107 This genodermatitis shown in the sternal skin is often widespread and flexural; it usually starts at puberty.

(a) What are its eponymous and official names?

(b) What is its mode of inheritance?

(c) Name some associated systemic disorders?

108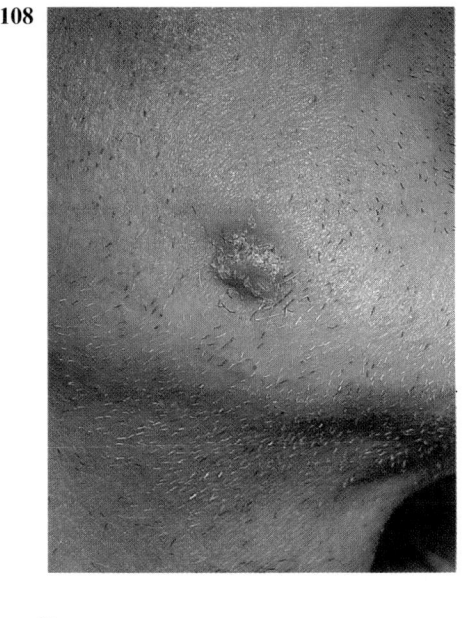

108 This elderly man had a discharging lesion over the right mandible for about 6 months.

(a) What is the probable diagnosis?

(b) How would you prove the diagnosis?

(c) What is the treatment?

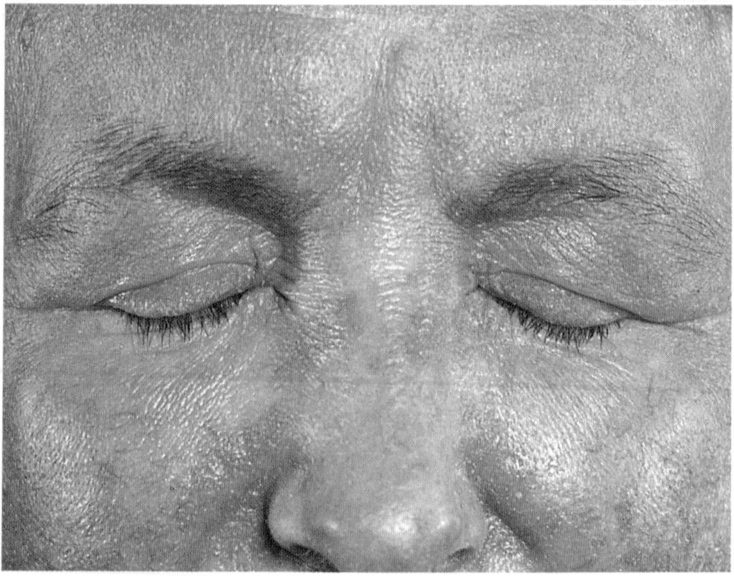

109

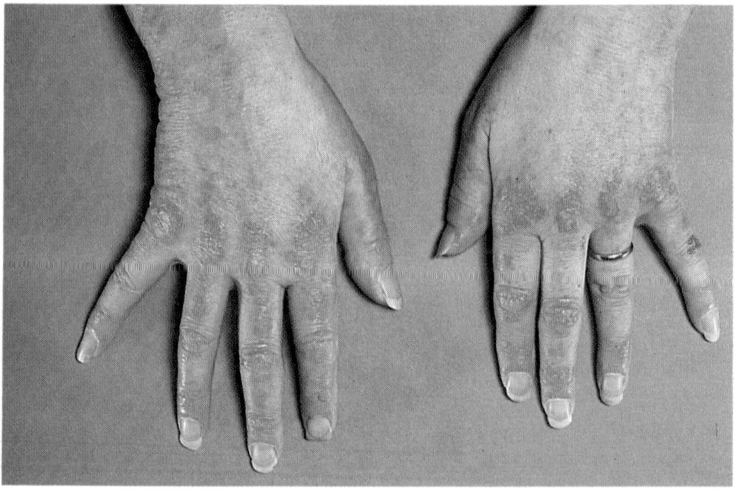

110

109, 110 This eruption occurred in a middle-aged lady.
(a) How would you describe the physical signs?
(b) What general symptoms should you ask about?
(c) What is the diagnosis?
(d) What important associated problem may be present?

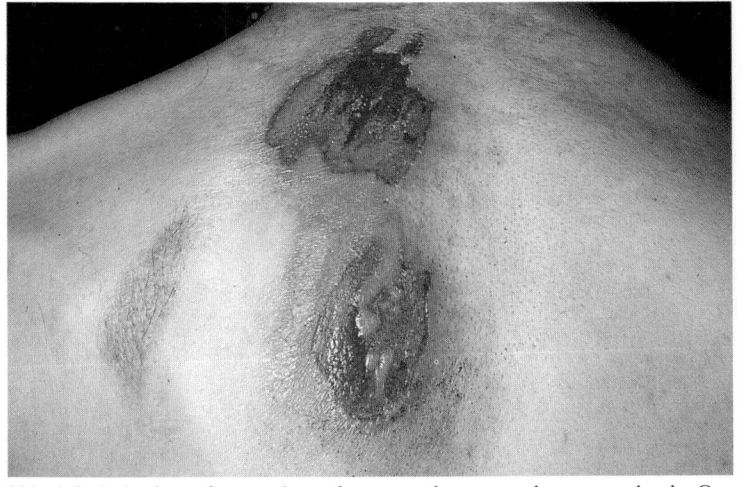

111 A lady had persistent ulcers for several years on her upper back. One has healed with scarring.
(a) What are the ulcers?
(b) What is the differential diagnosis?
(c) What is the prognosis?

112 A young woman had a 10-day history of tender red lumps on the legs.
(a) What is the diagnosis?
(b) How many possible causes can you suggest?

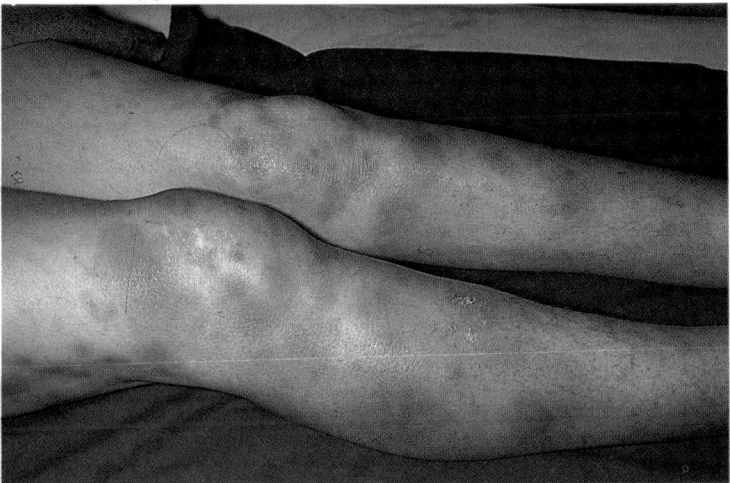

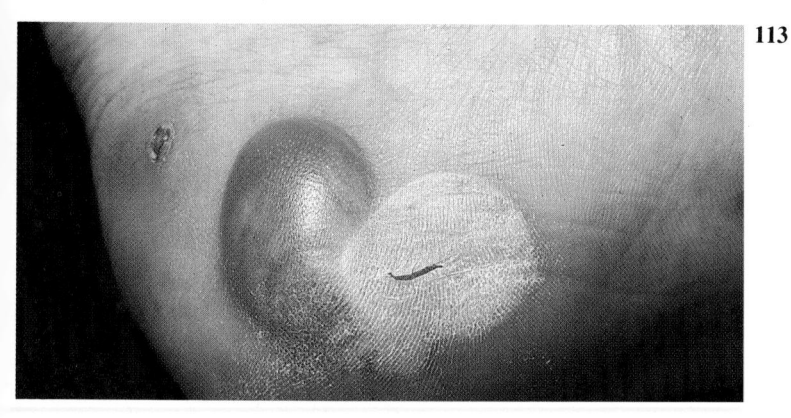

113 A teenager had recurrent blisters of the heels and soles; her mother had been similarly affected at the same age.
(a) What is the likely diagnosis?
(b) From what should you differentiate it?

114 There is an itchy marginated scaly pink eruption on the foot and ankle.
(a) What is it?
(b) What investigations are needed?

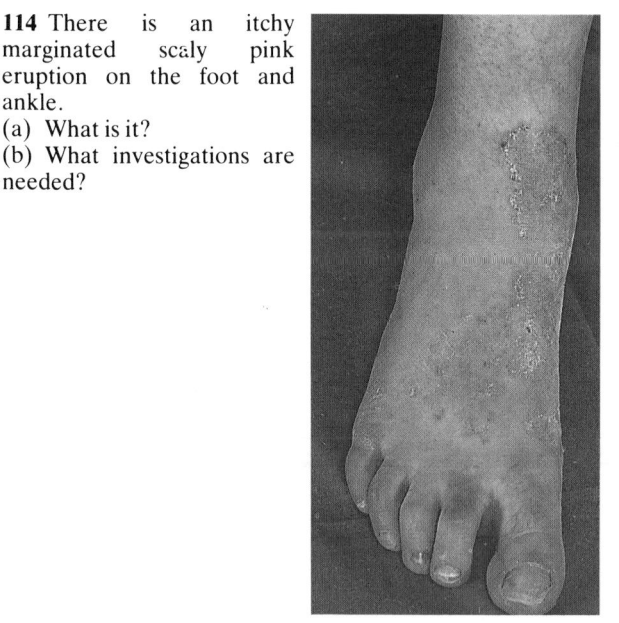

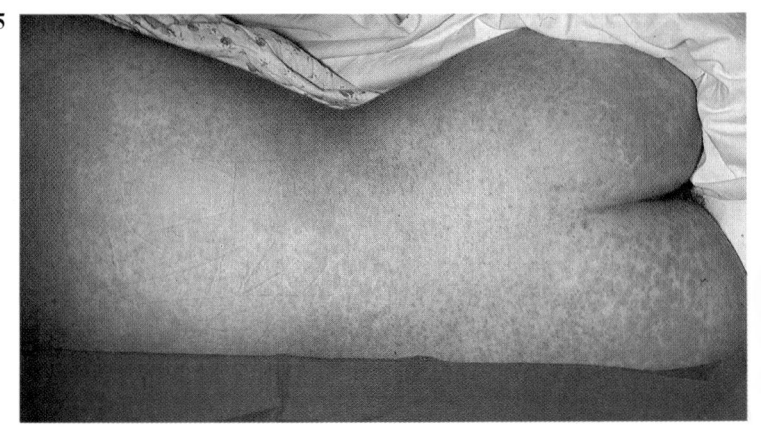

115 A young woman presented with fever, sore throat and enlarged lymph nodes when she developed this profuse maculo-papular eruption.
(a) What is the likely diagnosis?
(b) What other physical signs would you look for to confirm the diagnosis?

116 There is a pigmented eruption over the child's body. The lesions form weals if rubbed.
(a) What is the cause?
(b) Where are internal lesions of the condition found?
(c) What is the prognosis?

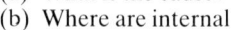
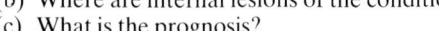
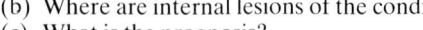
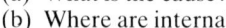
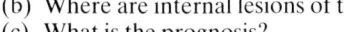
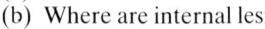
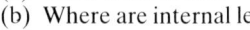
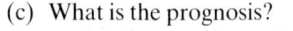
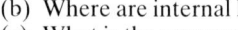

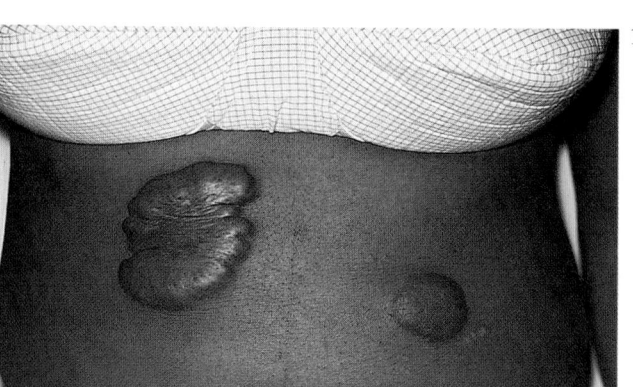

117 In this African lady, hard plaques formed at the site of severe insect bites sustained several years previously.

(a) What are they?
(b) What else may produce them?
(c) What symptoms are likely?
(d) What happens if they are surgically excised?

118 This lady was referred from the Haematology department when she developed a purplish nodular eruption on both arms.

(a) What are the nodules likely to be caused by?
(b) What was the original diagnosis?

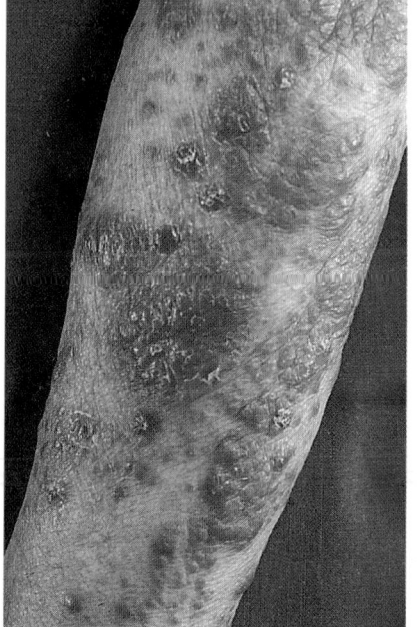

119

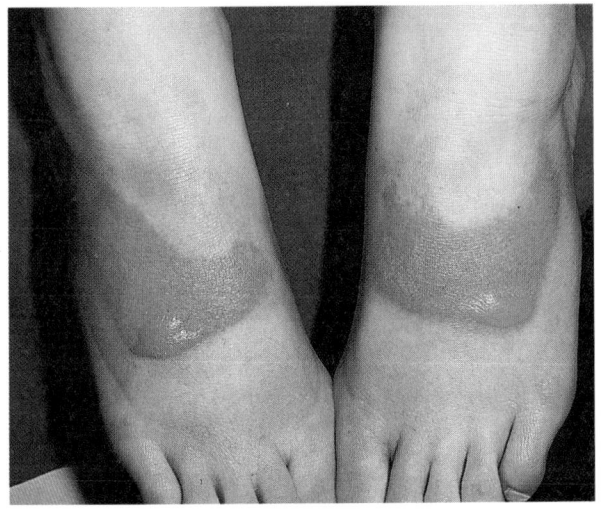

119 A lady developed blisters on her feet after sitting in her garden in the summer; she was recovering from a urinary infection.
(a) What had happened?
(b) Name 3 other conditions which sunlight may exacerbate.

120 (a) What is this lesion which was present at birth?
(b) What underlying condition can occur?
(c) Is there any complication of the skin lesion?

120

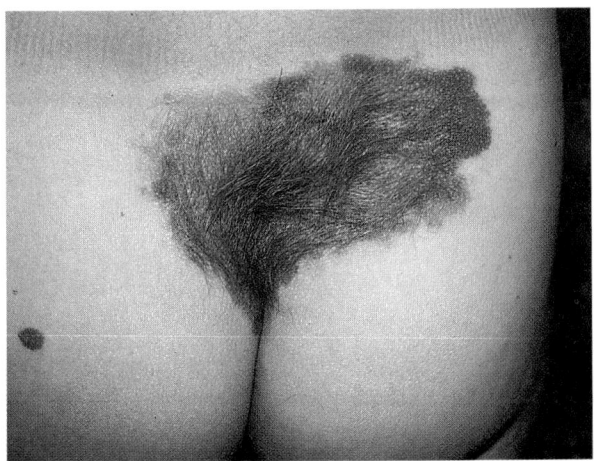

121 The patient had a ten-year history of increasing numbers of pruritic brownish-red scaly plaques developing on her hips and elsewhere on the body. She does not have psoriasis.

(a) What is the diagnosis?
(b) How would you confirm the diagnosis?
(c) What is the prognosis?

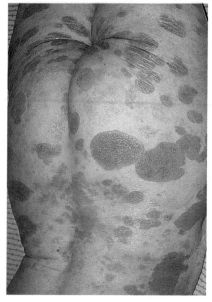

122 This man is of Indian origin and most of his family show normal Indian pigmentation.

(a) What is wrong with him?
(b) What is the genetic background to the disorder?
(c) Why is regular follow-up necessary?

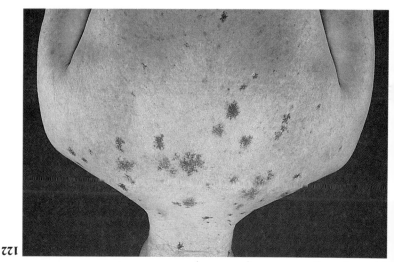

123 This symmetrical, occasionally pruritic, widespread eruption had been present for about a week.

(a) What is it?
(b) What skin sign might have preceded it?
(c) How long will it last?

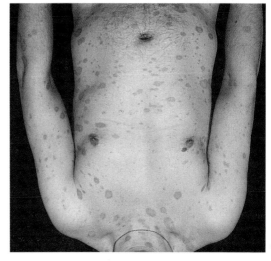

124 (a) How do you account for the pale patches on this man's neck and chest?
(b) What is the differential diagnosis?

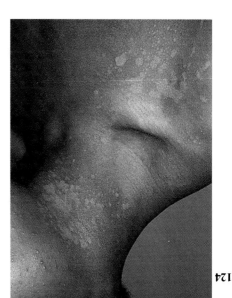

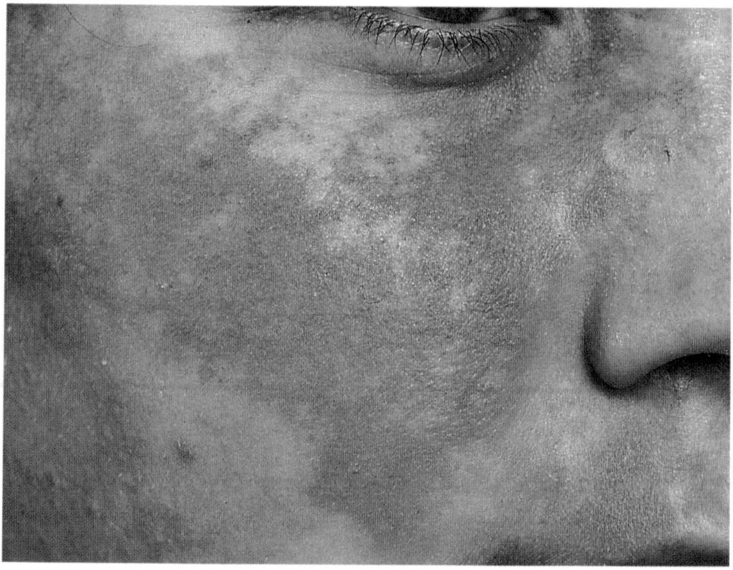

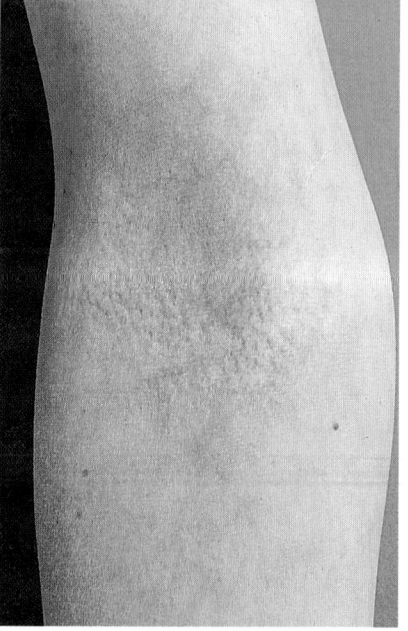

125 (a) What is this lesion which was present from birth?
(b) With which syndrome is it sometimes associated?

126 A lady, aged 35 years, had suffered two episodes of melaena. On admission to hospital she had this unusual appearance of her elbow flexures.
(a) What is the skin disorder called?
(b) Where else on the skin would you look for similar lesions?
(c) How is it related to her episodes of malaena?
(d) What other systemic disorders may occur?

127

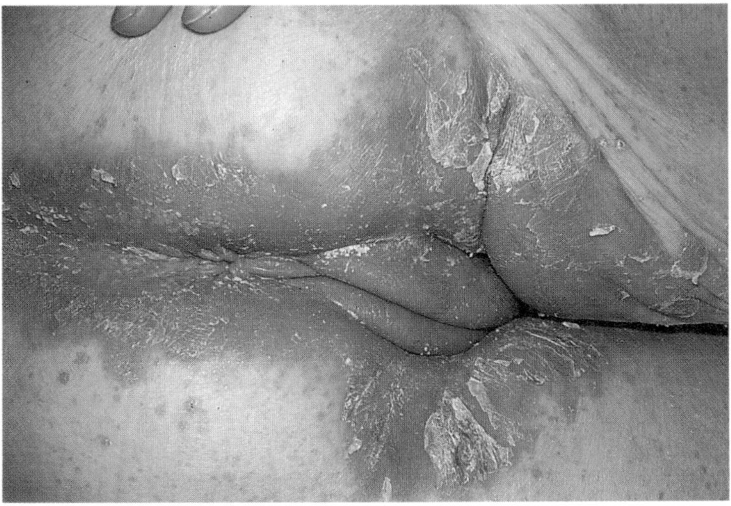

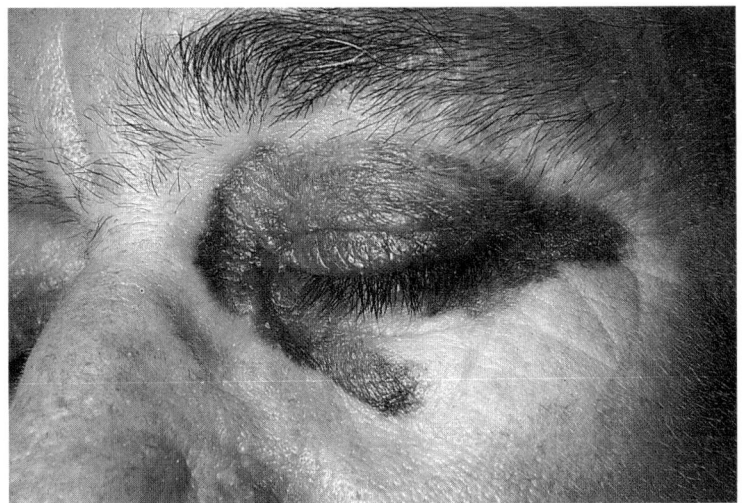

127 This lady had anogenital pruritus.
(a) What is the problem?
(b) From what should it be distinguished?

128 What skin infiltration can lead to this eyelid haemorrhage, which occurred without trauma?

128

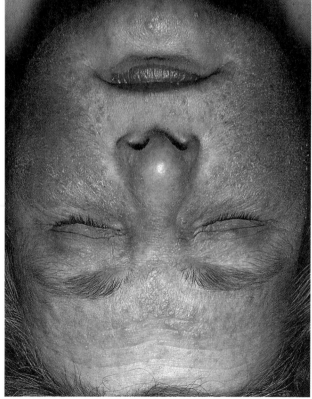

129 This lady had a mildly uncomfortable pustular eruption over the face for several months.

(a) What is it?
(b) What other symptoms would you ask about?
(c) How is it best treated?

130 A middle-aged man complained of painful ears, both of which showed similar inflammation.
(a) What is the diagnosis and how can you be confident of it clinically?
(b) Which two investigations would be helpful?
(c) Where else may lesions be found?

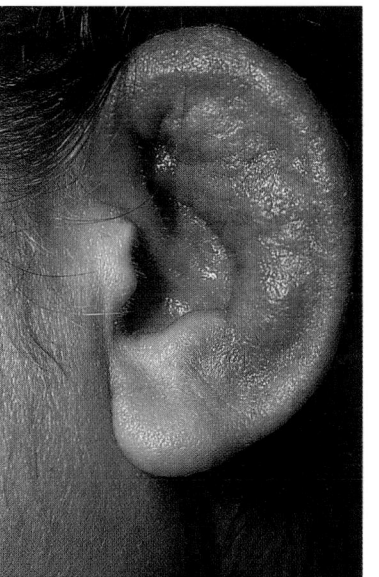

131 (a) What is causing the hard, painless finger swellings?
(b) What would an X-ray show?

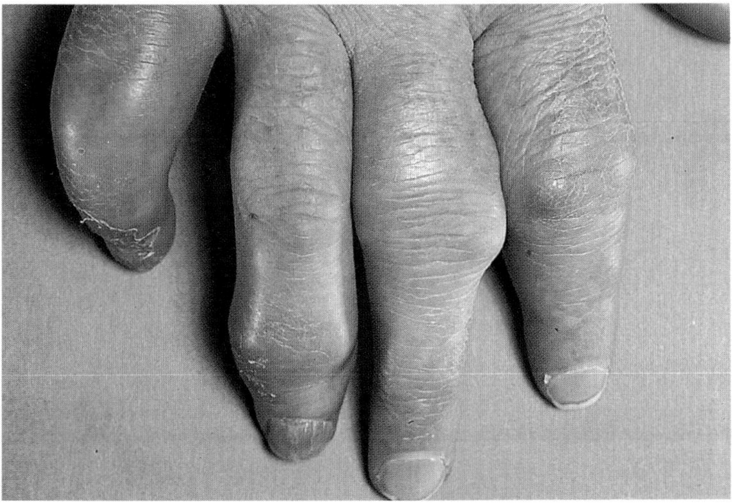

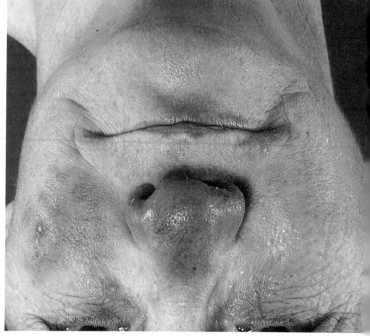

132 (a) What is the cause of this lady's blue nose?
(b) What differential diagnoses should be considered?

133 (a) What is this arthropod?
(b) What symptoms and signs does it cause?
(c) Where does it lay its eggs?
(d) How is it eliminated?

134

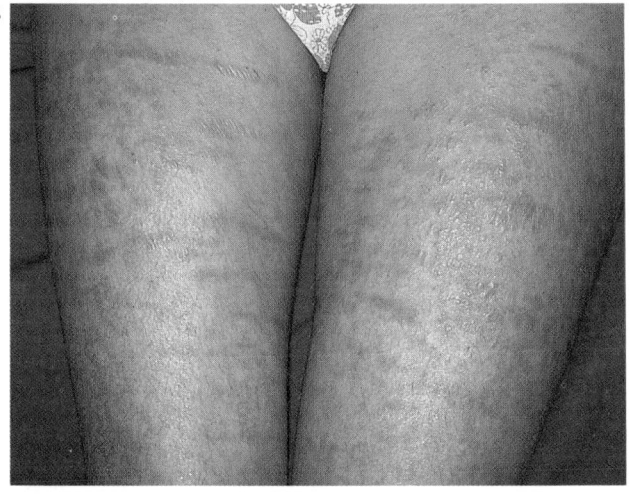

134 What are these lesions and how were they caused?

135 The lesion on the lower lip of this elderly man grew without symptoms for several months.
(a) What is the likely diagnosis?
(b) How would you prove it?
(c) What is the most important factor in its production?

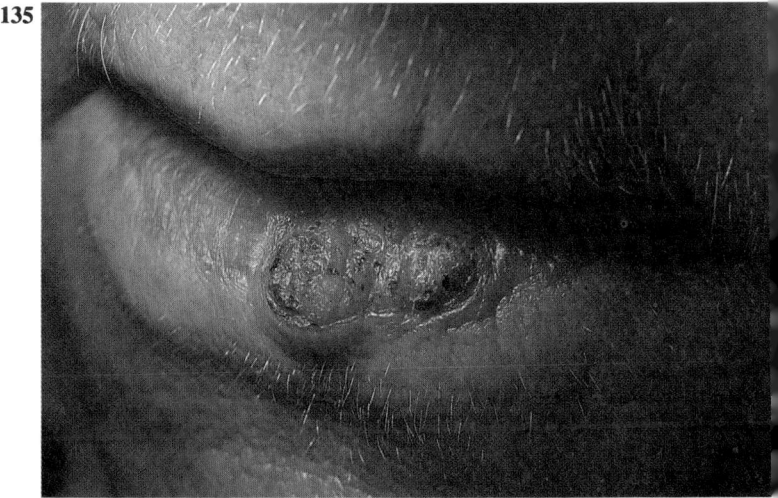

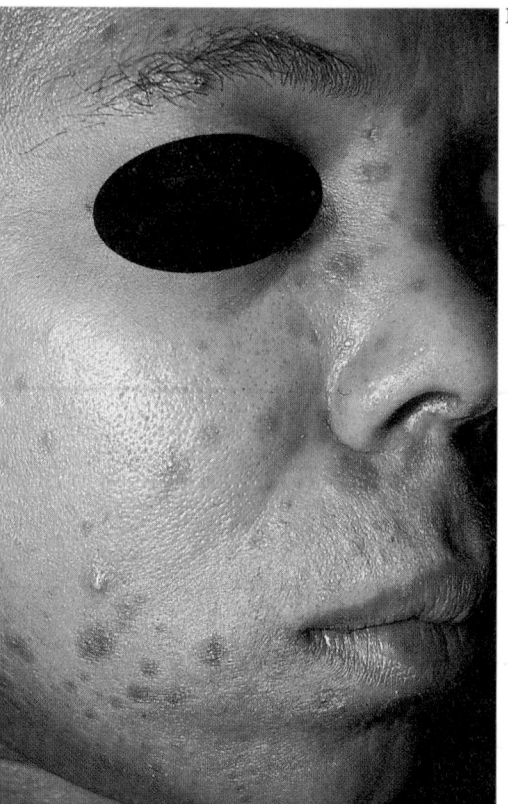

136 The patient had a symptomless eruption on her face for several weeks and felt unwell. She had cervical and epitrochlear lymphadenopathy.
(a) What is the likely diagnosis?
(b) What blood test would be helpful?

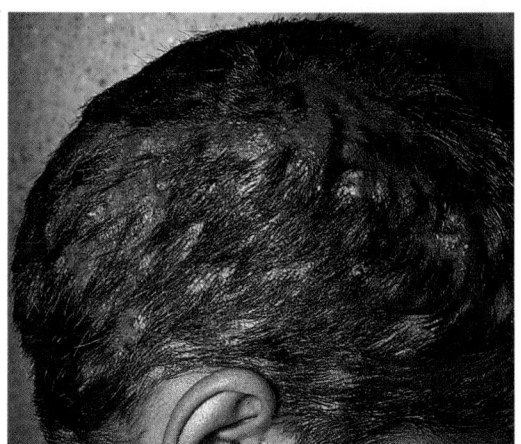

137 A child's irregular patchy hair loss had been made worse with topical corticosteroid ointment.
(a) What is the cause of the alopecia?
(b) What investigations are desirable?
(c) What is the best treatment?

138 A 75-year-old Greek lady had a five-year history of increasing purple-brown non-pruritic purpuric plaques on the legs.
(a) What are they?
(b) In whom are they found?
(c) What is the differential diagnosis?
(d) What is the prognosis?

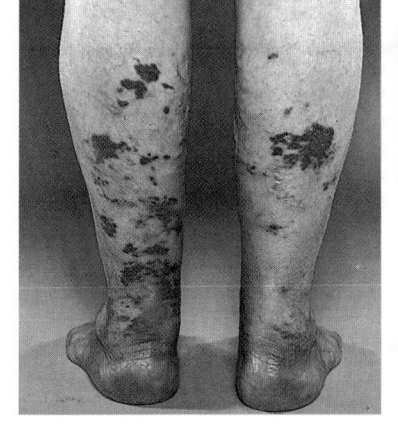

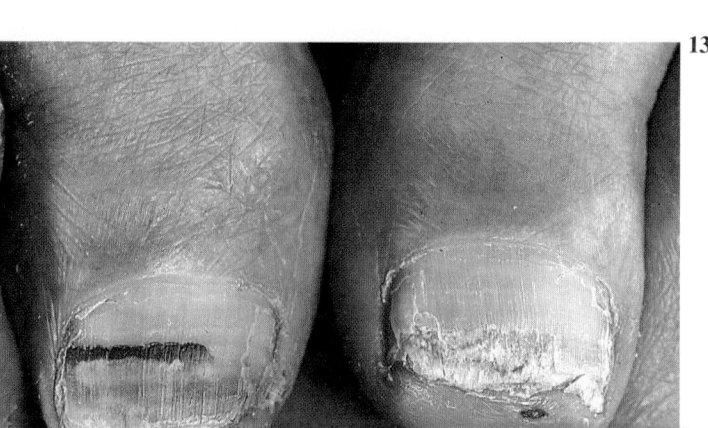

139 (a) What may cause these thickened friable hallux nails?
(b) What investigations could help diagnosis?
(c) Why is there a transverse haemorrhage in the right hallux nail?

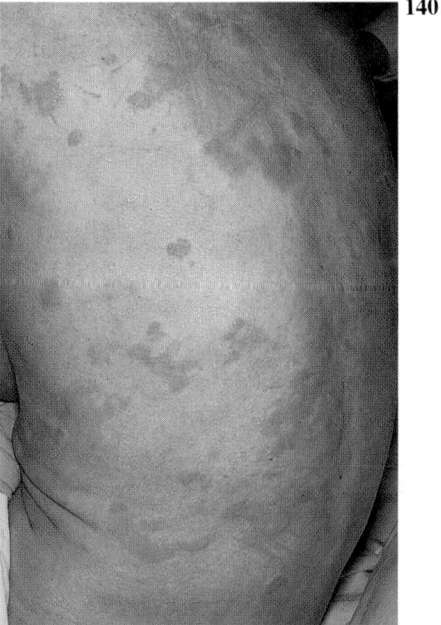

140 The patient had a daily changing eruption of itchy weals.
(a) What is the diagnosis?
(b) What varieties of the condition are encountered?
(c) How is it best treated?

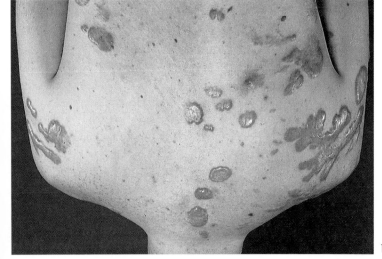

141 (a) What has caused the keloid scars on this young man's back?

(b) How can they be treated?

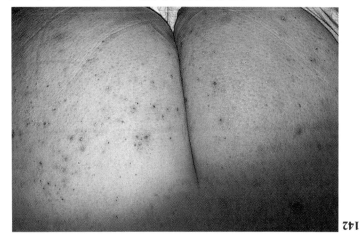

142, 143, 144 (a) What single disease is shown?

(b) What is illustrated?

(c) How is the disease acquired?

(d) How is it treated?

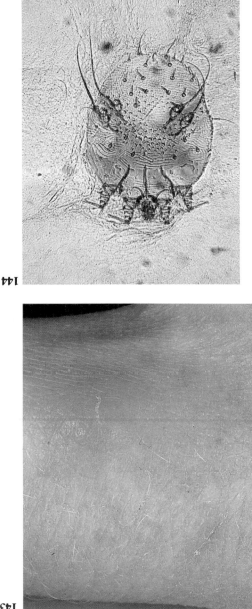

144

143

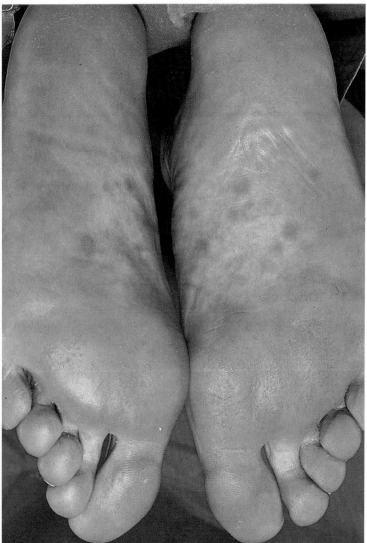

145 This man was on a medical ward with fever, malaise and lymph-adenopathy. A provisional diagnosis of Hodgkin's disease was made; an eruption was then noticed.
(a) What is the correct diagnosis?
(b) Where else would you look for lesions?

145

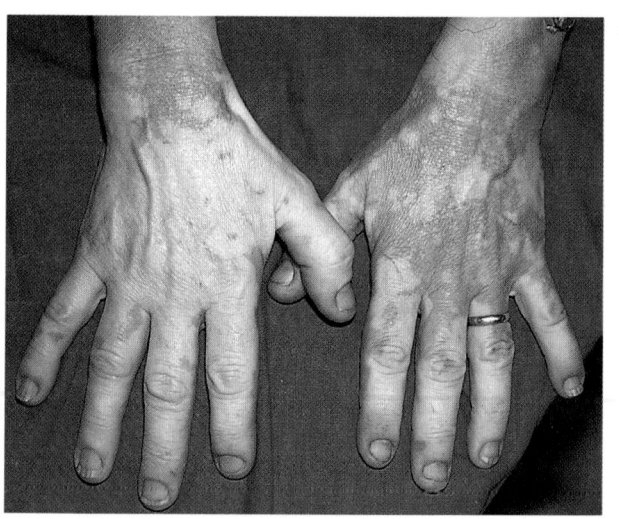

146 A man had symmetrical depigmentation affecting his limbs and trunk.
(a) What is the disorder?
(b) With what systemic disease may it be associated?
(c) Is an external cause ever responsible?
(d) What is the syndrome in which this disorder is associated with bilateral uveitis, deafness, loss of hair pigment and alopecia areata.

147 A 4mm lesion on the thigh was one of several on the limbs and trunk which indicated a rare and potentially lethal disease.
(a) What is the diagnosis?
(b) How may it terminate?

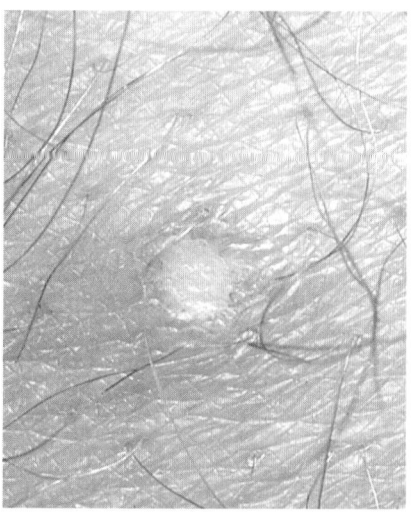

147

148 (a) What is the eruption of small papules on this man's face?
(b) List the causes of papular lesions on the face.

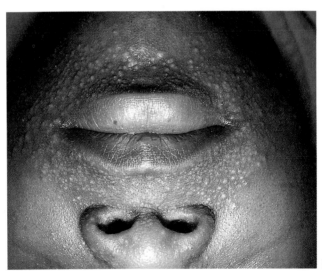

148

149 A 21-year-old girl presented with a one week history of tender nodules on her fingers, a painful swollen left wrist and a fever of 38°C.
(a) What is the likely diagnosis?
(b) How may it be confirmed?

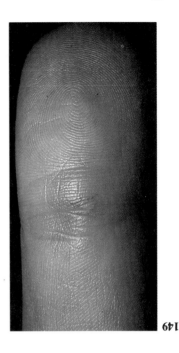

149

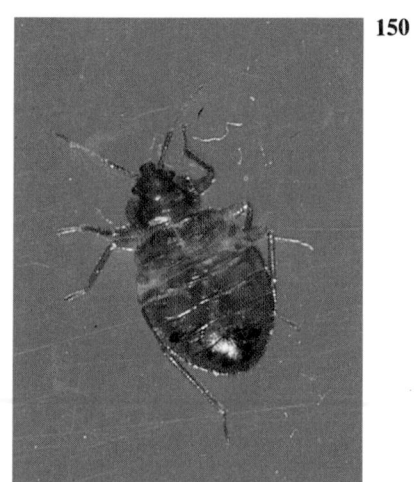

150, 151 An insect which is about 4mm long, caused these lesions.
(a) What is it?
(b) How does it find its host?

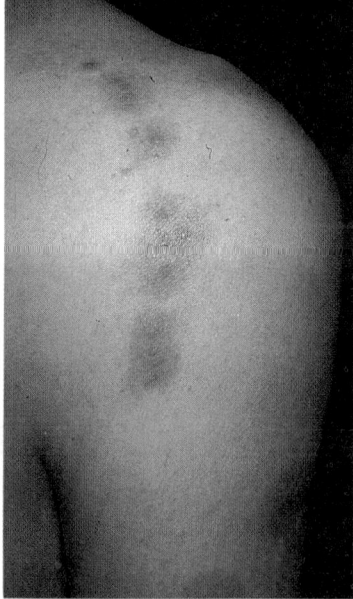

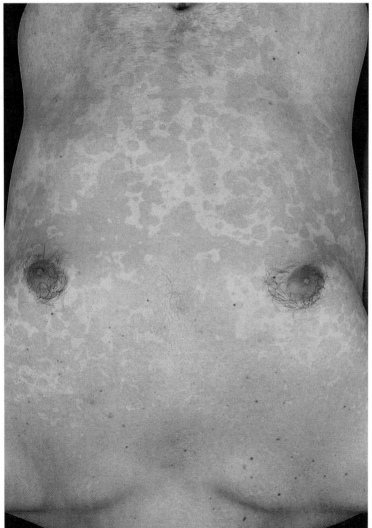

152

152 A symptomless, pink, slightly scaly eruption increased throughout 3 years over a man's trunk.

(a) What is it?
(b) What is the cause?
(c) How would you treat it?

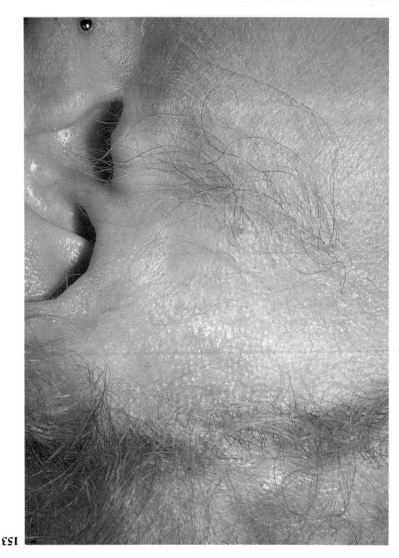

153 An otherwise well lady complained of increasing loss of hair on both sides of her scalp.

(a) What might have caused this?
(b) What is the prognosis?

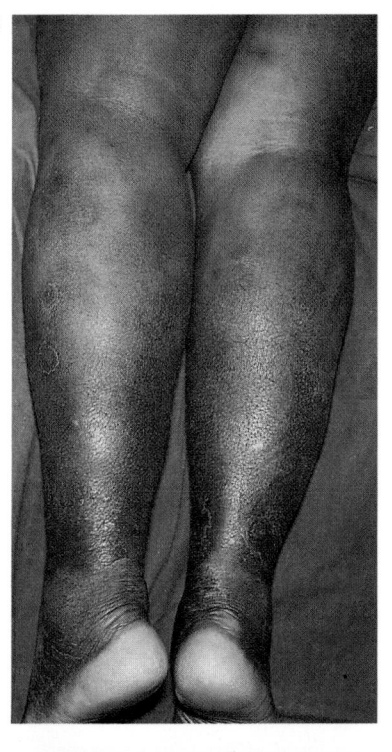

154 This 45-year-old lady had persistent tender deep plaques symmetrically in her calves; her Mantoux test was strongly positive at 1:10,000.
(a) What is the diagnosis?
(b) What other investigations are needed?
(c) How should it be treated?

155 This man complained of itchy eyelids.
(a) What is the reason?
(b) What is the more usual site for this problem?

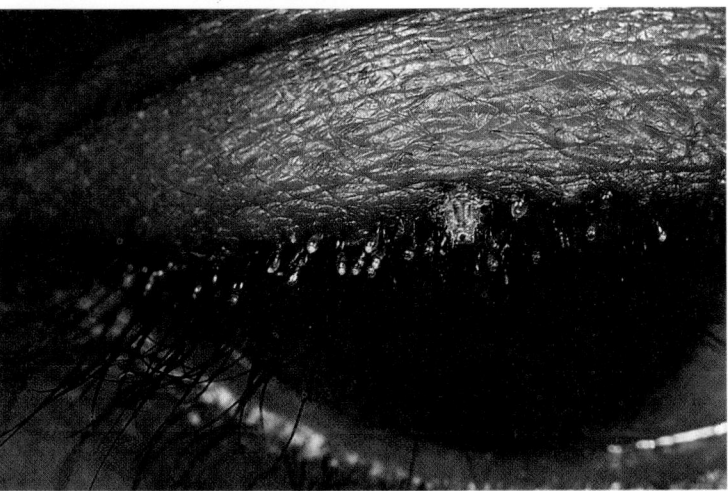

156 A man had a six months' history of painless nodules growing on the dorsum of his right little finger. His (indoor) hobby gave the clue to the correct diagnosis.

(a) What are the nodules?
(b) What was his hobby?
(c) What is the organism?
(d) What would you include in the differential diagnosis?

157 Why does this man have a painful blue hallux?

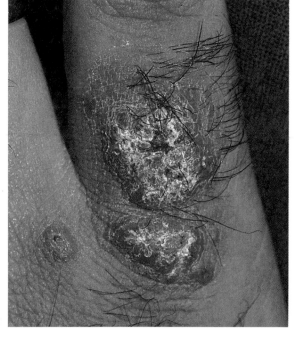

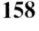

158 An acutely ill young woman was admitted with a fever and a wide-spread erythematous and pustular eruption.
(a) What is it?
(b) From what must it be distinguished?
(c) How is it usually treated?

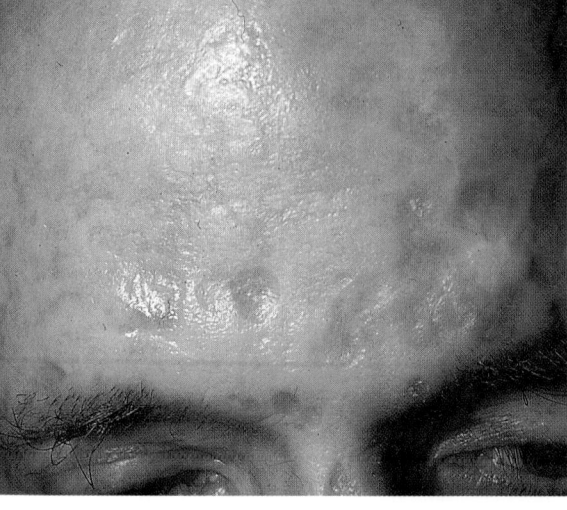

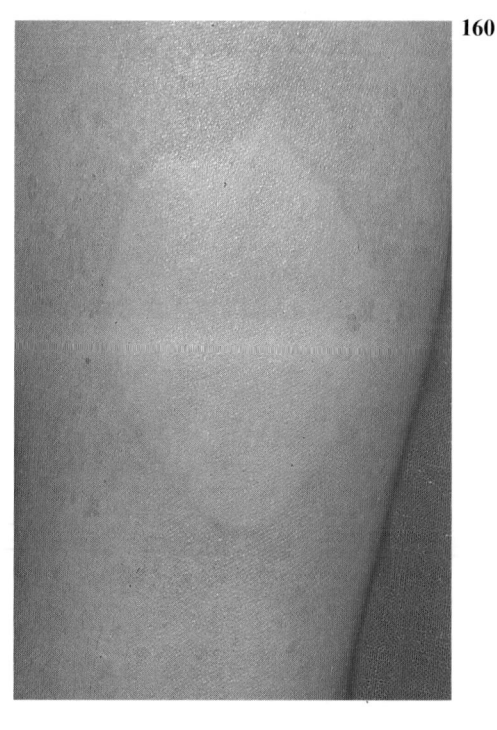

159 An elderly man had a two-year history of blisters developing on his forehead and which healed to form scars.
(a) What is wrong with him?
(b) What might have precipitated the condition?
(c) What investigations would confirm the diagnosis?

160 This appearance was produced by a 2-minute application of an ice cube to the forearm. The procedure confirmed the clinical diagnosis.
(a) What is the diagnosis?
(b) List some other conditions which may be provoked by cold.

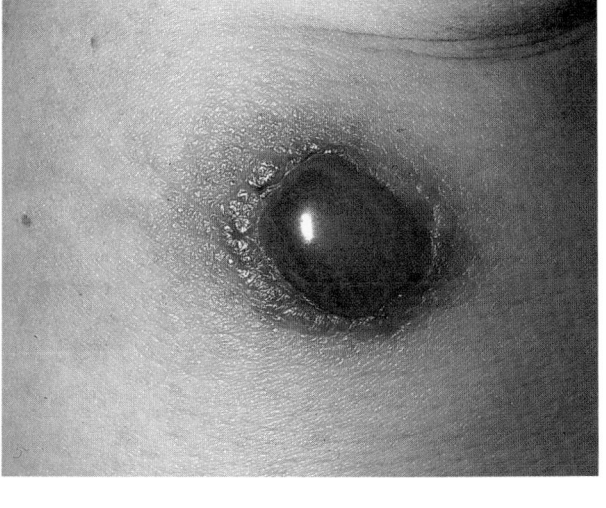

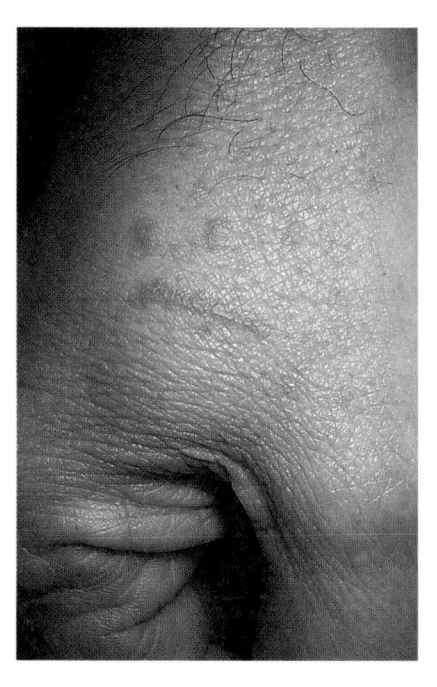

161 While being treated for leukaemia, this ill man developed several large blisters on a necrotic base.
(a) What had happened?
(b) What other cutaneous manifestations of leukaemia do you recognise?

162 This man had lichen planus. During the course of the disease he developed a linear lesion in a scratch on the dorsum of his hand.
(a) What is this phenomenon called?
(b) What other skin disorders may behave in this way?

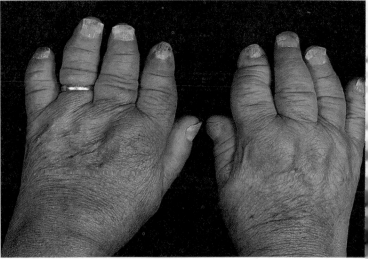

164 Why does this lady have such deformed hands?

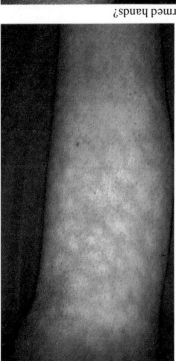

163 This is the left lower leg of a man with a symmetrical net-like cyanotic erythema on his legs.

(a) What is this condition?
(b) What gives rise to it?

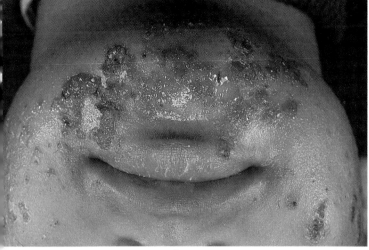

166 This young man had a spreading exudative and crusted eruption on his chin for 10 days.
  (a) What is the eruption?
  (b) What organisms are responsible?
  (c) What internal disease is a rare complication?

166

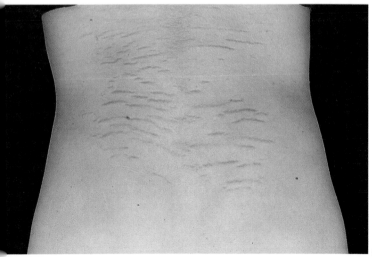

165 What are the lines on this young man's back?

165

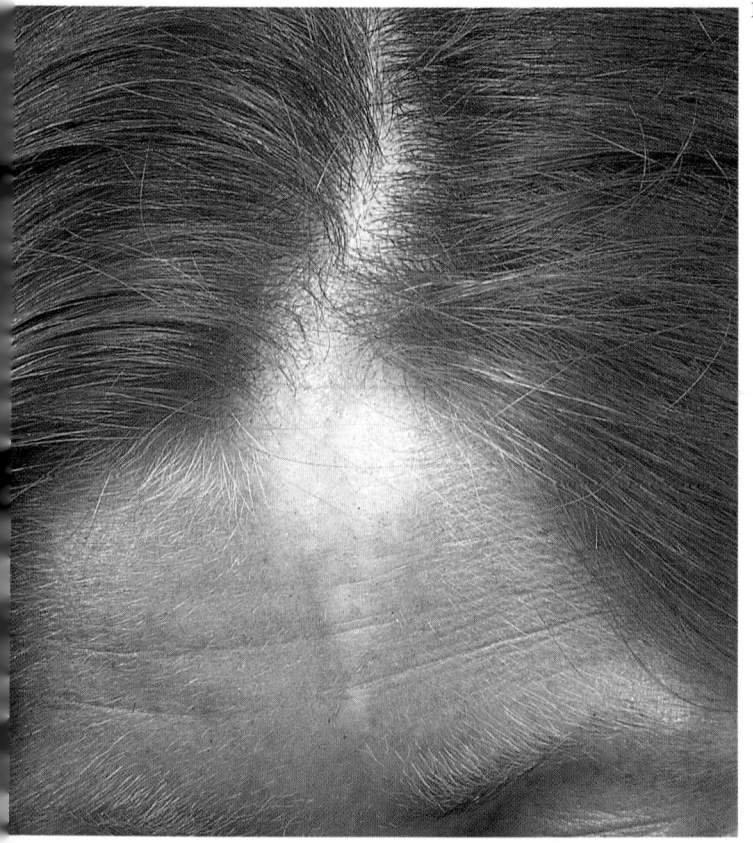

167 A young woman has a white sclerotic plaque with hair loss at the frontal margin which has gradually extended down her forehead.
(a) What is this condition?
(b) How could it progress?
(c) What complications may be associated with it?

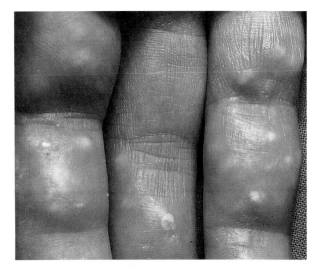

168 (a) Why does this man's dermatitis stop at the line of his collar?
(b) What therapy may produce a similar reaction?

169 (a) What are the tender white nodules on this lady's fingers?
(b) In which disorders may they be found?

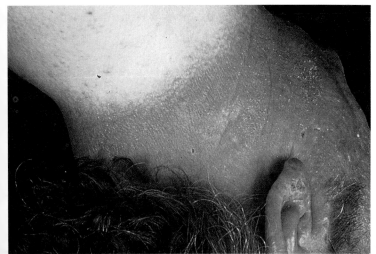

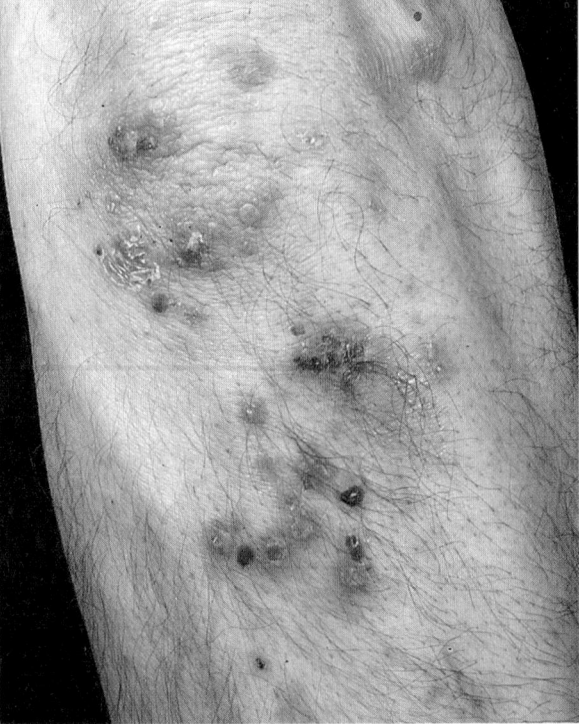

170 A man had a six months' history of a very itchy symmetrical eruption of vesicles and crusts on his elbows and elsewhere; his left elbow, with drying vesicles and excoriations is shown.

(a) What is the likely diagnosis?

(b) With which internal disorder is it associated?

(c) Where else should one look for lesions?

(d) From which other itchy skin disorder must it be differentiated?

(e) How is it treated?

171 This elderly lady had progressively darkening skin for two years. She was found to have an enlarged liver and sugar in her urine.
(a) What is the likely diagnosis?
(b) What investigations confirm the diagnosis?
(c) What other systemic disorders give rise to cutaneous hyperpigmentation?

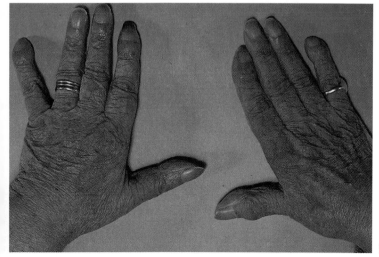

171

172 This lady had symptomless discoloration of her axillae for about 5 years and her groins were also affected.
(a) What is the diagnosis?
(b) With which systemic disorder is it frequently found?
(c) Which two investigations are used to confirm the diagnosis?

172

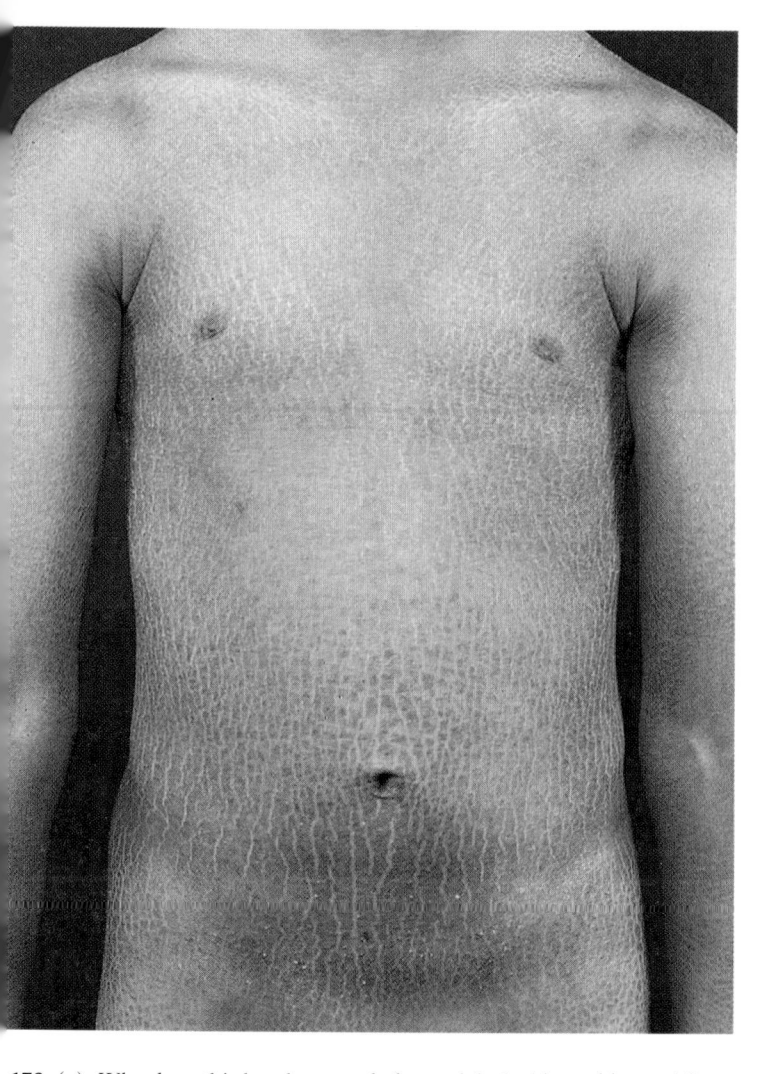

173 (a) Why does this boy have such dry and dark skin on his trunk?
(b) List some systemic diseases which may induce a dry skin.

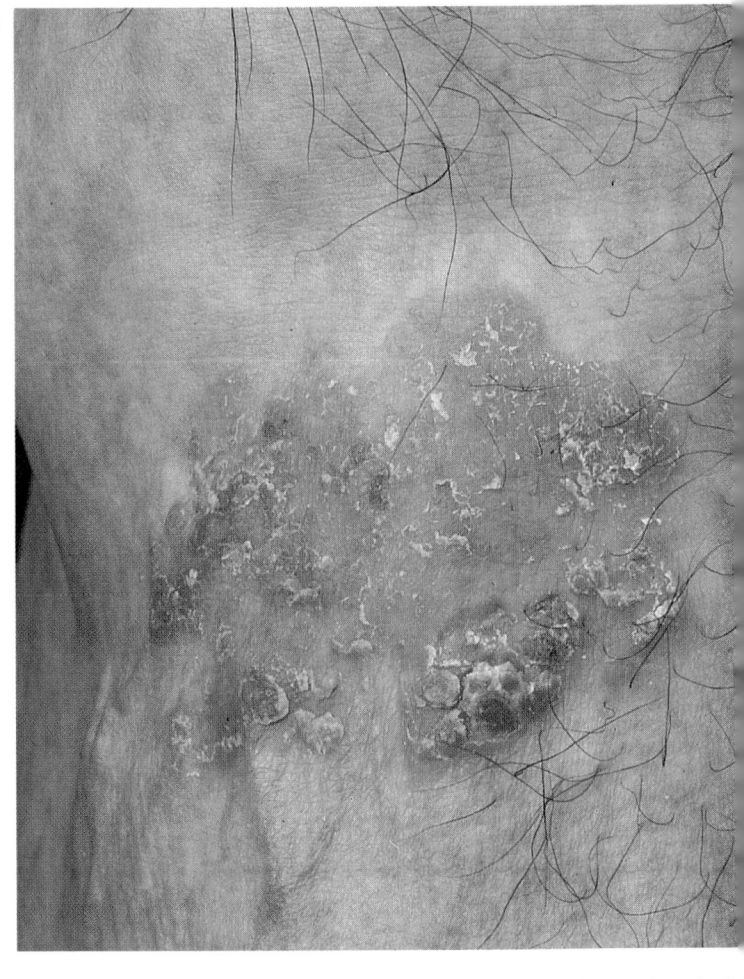

174 A middle-aged man had a five-year history of a slowly growing single red plaque on the anterior aspect of his left ankle.
(a) What is it?
(b) What is the differential diagnosis?
(c) What happens to these lesions if they are not treated?

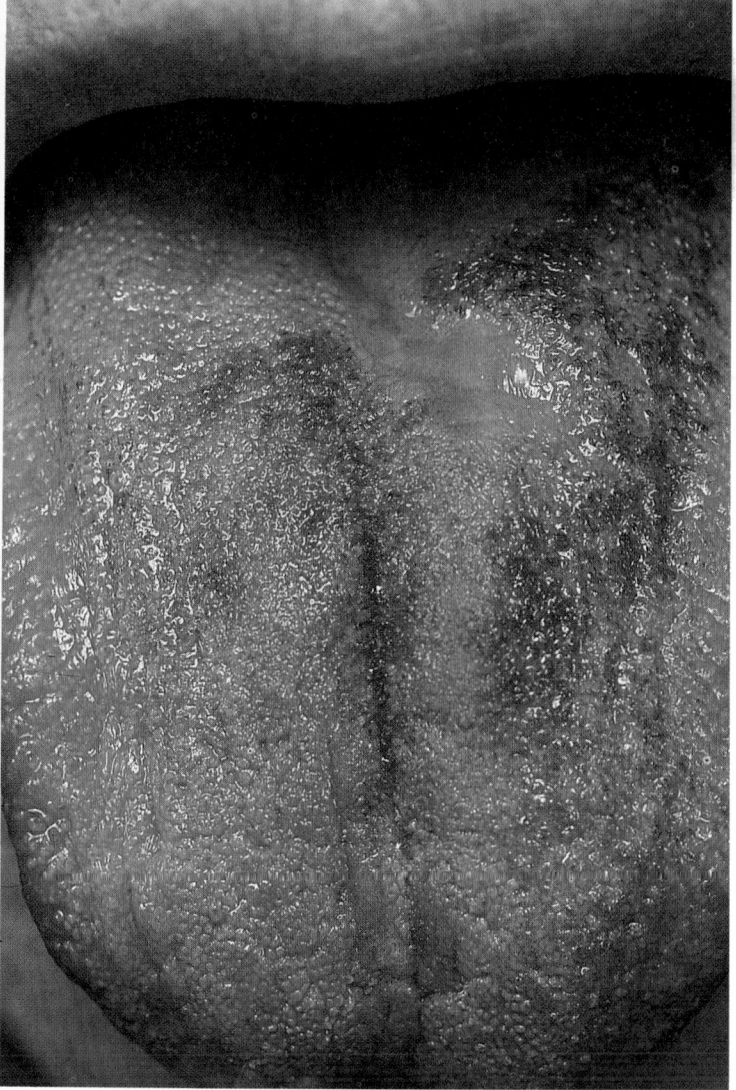

175 (a) What is wrong with this man's tongue?
(b) What can predispose to it?

176 A child had a changing pattern of slightly scaly slightly hypopigmented patches on his face.

(a) What is this condition?
(b) What is the prognosis?

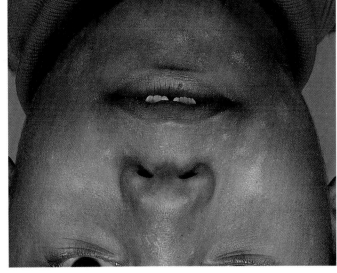

177 A young woman returned from a Mediterranean holiday complaining of painful finger-nails.

(a) What was she suffering from?
(b) What could have caused it?

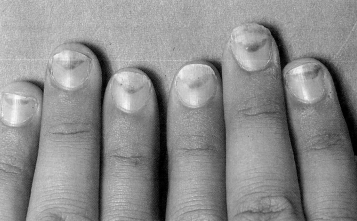

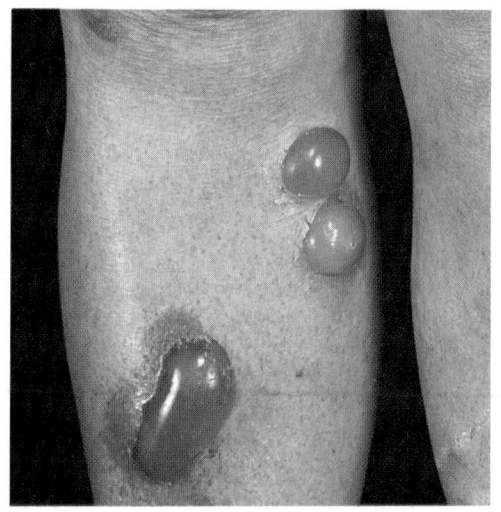

178 A group of itchy spots on this lady's legs two days before developed into large blisters. Otherwise well, no lesions were present above her knees.
(a) What are the lesions?
(b) How may they have been acquired?

179 (a) What is the cause of this lady's painful inflamed finger web which she has had for several months?
(b) What predisposes to the problem?

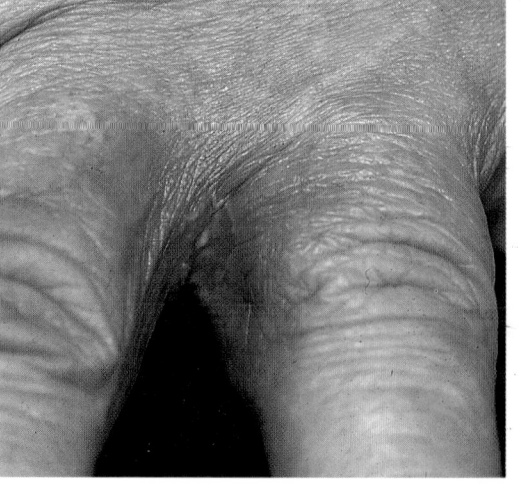

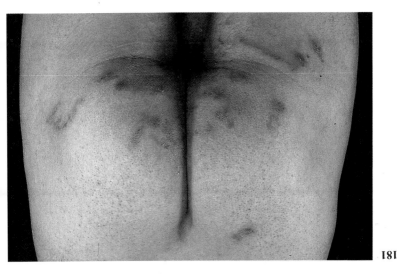

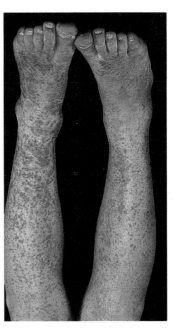

180 The child became unwell and developed abdominal pain, painful swelling of the joints and a purpuric eruption on the lower legs. Her platelet count was normal and she had received no drugs.
(a) What is this condition?
(b) What other problems might arise?
(c) What is the cause?

181 A few weeks after returning from a sub-tropical beach holiday, a man developed an intensely pruritic linear and arcuate eruption on the buttocks.
(a) What is it?
(b) What causes it?
(c) Is there any internal association?
(d) What is the prognosis?

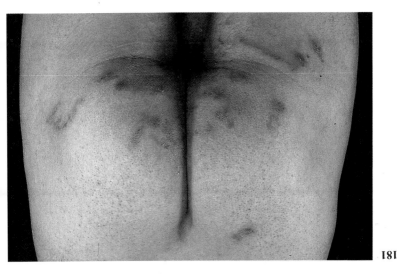

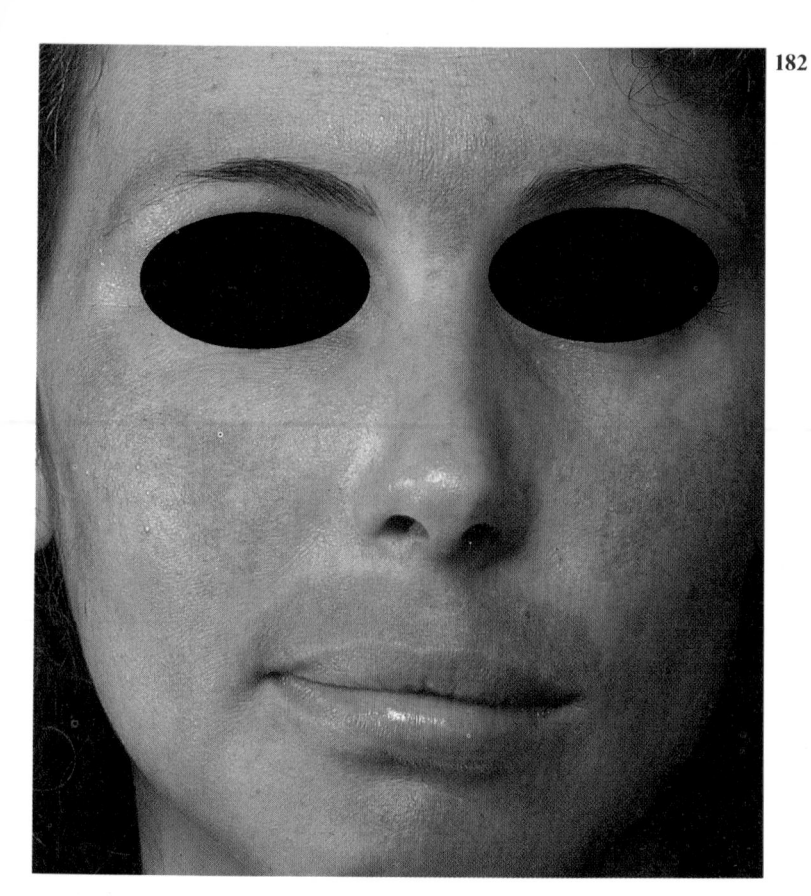

182 (a) What is the symmetrical hyperpigmentation on this lady's face?
(b) What may predispose to it?

183

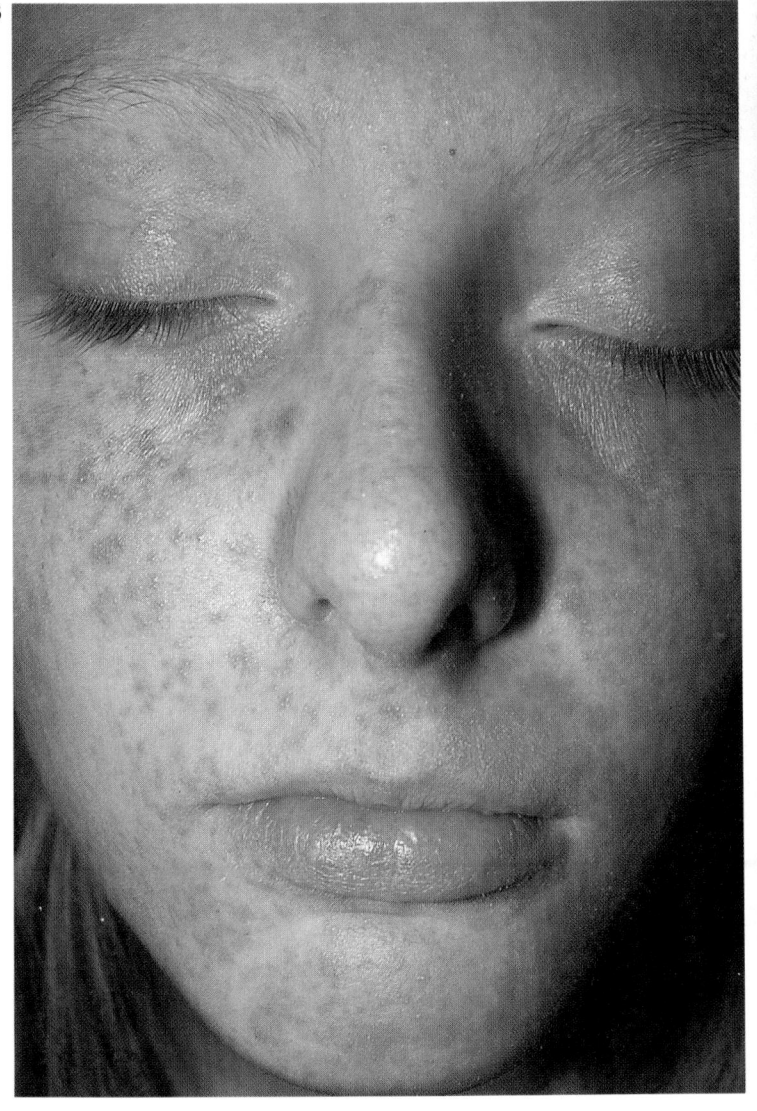

183 A girl had a few small spots on her chin and cheeks. The treatment she used for several months caused increasing redness and pustule formation.
(a) What had happened?
(b) How should she be treated now?

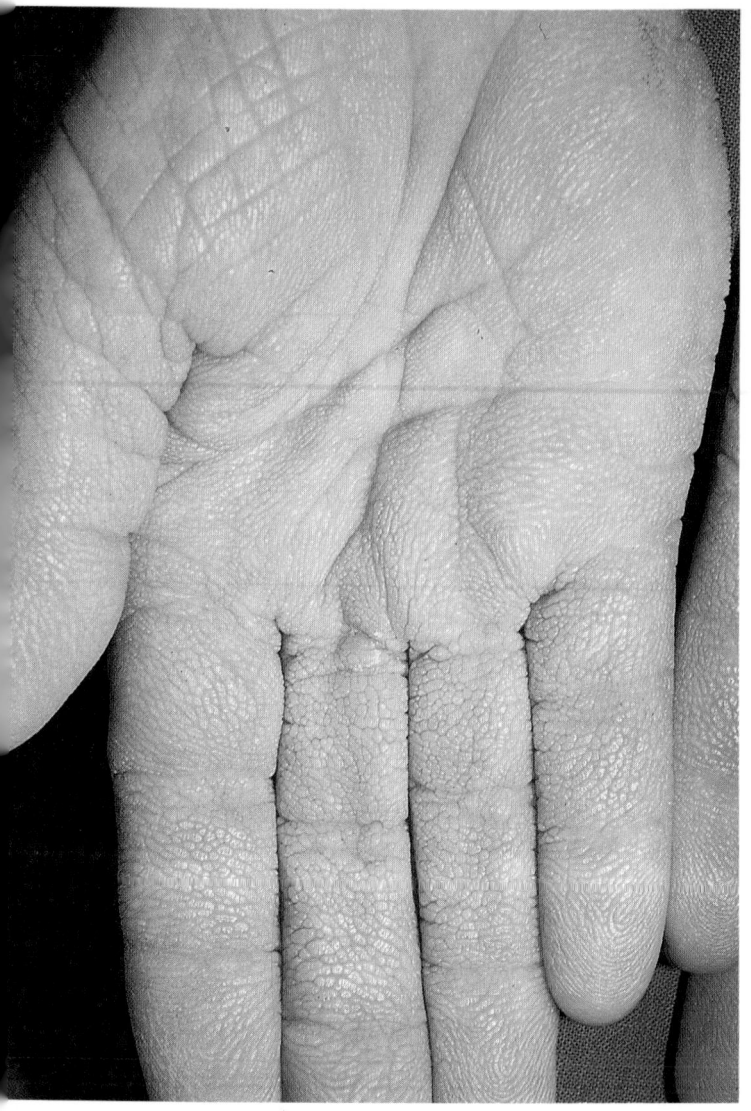

184 This man's palms and flexor aspect of his fingers show gross exaggeration of the ridge pattern.
(a) What is this appearance sometimes called?
(b) What is the diagnosis?
(c) What other lesions would you look for?
(d) Why is the condition important, even though very rare?

185 A 6-year-old girl had suffered with a chronic sore mouth, vulvo-vaginitis and this nail dystrophy since infancy.

(a) What rare disorder does she have?

(b) What other problems can be found in association?

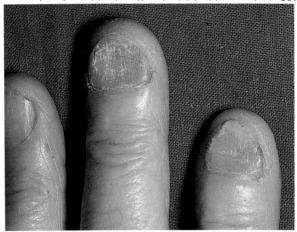

186

186 A 32-year-old woman presented with silvery plaques over the elbows. The affected areas were not itchy but gentle removal of the scales caused 'pinpoint' bleeding.

(a) What is the diagnosis?

(b) Where else should you look for lesions?

(c) With what may it be associated?

185

ANSWERS

1 (a) Pyogenic granuloma – often a result of trauma. Patient's occupation exposes the fingers to injury often unnoticed.
(b) Amelanotic melanoma. The lesion after removal should be sent for histological examination.
(c) Curettage and diathermy under local anaesthetic.

2 (a) Necrobiosis lipoidica associated with diabetes mellitus.
(b) Ulceration of a necrobiotic plaque is not infrequent.
(c) Erythema nodosum; diabetic dermopathy; pretibial myxoedema.

3 (a) Bullous pemphigoid.
(b) Biopsy of a fresh blister for routine histology and immunofluorescent studies on perilesional skin. Skin adjacent to a fresh lesion less than 12 hours old is best examined.
(c) Dermatitis herpetiformis, pemphigus vulgaris, bullous erythema multiforme, epidermolysis bullosa, bullous impetigo, porphyria cutanea tarda.

4 (a) Pemphigus vulgaris.
(b) Large doses of systemic corticosteroids, usually with immunosuppressive drugs – azathioprine, cyclophosphamide or methotrexate – which act as steroid sparing agents.

5 (a) Herpes zoster.
(b) Thoracic dermatomes (53%), next most common are cervical dermatomes usually C2, 3 and 4 (20%).
(c) Secondary bacterial infection; scarring; post-herpetic neuralgia.

6 (a) Herpes simplex.
(b) Direct inoculation of the virus into the abrasion.
(c) Viral culture of blister fluid.

7 (a) Stevens-Johnson syndrome.
(b) The eyes, in 90 per cent of cases.
(c) The commonest associations are with preceding herpes simplex or Mycoplasma infection; also streptococcal infections and drug hypersensitivity.

8 (a) Cutaneous metastasis from recurrence of breast cancer.
(b) Biopsy of the lesion for histopathology.
(c) Basal cell carcinoma.

9 (a) Lichen planus.
(b) Gold, organic mercurials, mepacrine, chloroquine, methyldopa, chlorpropamide, tolbutamide, quinidine; topical contact with colour film developer.

10 (a) Paget's disease of the breast invariably associated with an intraductal mammary carcinoma.
(c) Loss of the nipple.

11 (a) Herpes gestationis.
(b) Pruritus; pruritic urticarial papules; prurigo; impetigo herpetiformis (i.e. generalised pustular psoriasis).

12, 13 (a) Toxic epidermal necrolysis ('Lyell's disease' or 'scalded skin syndrome' from the appearance of the skin similar to that induced by a burn).
(b) They include drugs, particularly sulphonamides, barbiturates, allopurinol and phenytoin; cutaneous staphylococcal infection (*Staph-aureus*, phage type 71); miscellaneous – graft versus host reaction, exposure to petroleum distillates.

14 (a) Pyoderma gangrenosum. It tends to occur commonly on the lower limbs or trunk.
(b) Ulcerative colitis; Crohn's disease; chronic active hepatitis; rheumatoid arthritis; acute and chronic myeloid leukaemia; polycythaemia rubra vera; multiple myeloma, and monoclonal gammopathy (especially IgA).

15 (a) Pretibial myxoedema.
(b) Clinical signs of thyrotoxicosis. The skin may show vitiligo or diffuse hyper-pigmentation. There may be diffuse alopecia or clubbing of the fingers and toes with soft tissue swelling (i.e. thyroid acropathy). Onycholysis may occur and in some urticaria may be the presenting sign.
(c) Fluorinated corticosteroids applied under polythene occlusion to the pretibial plaques help in clearing the lesions.

16, 17 (a) Malignant melanoma.
(b) Seborrhoeic keratosis, compound melanocytic naevus, blue naevus, pigmented histiocytoma, pigmented basal cell carcinoma.
(c) Sheets of neoplastic melanocytes invading the dermis.

18 (a) Alopecia areata. The grey hairs have regrown in a previously bald patch.
(b) Vitiligo. Vitiligo and alopecia areata occur in association with uveitis in the Vogt-Koyanagi-Harada syndrome.
(c) Systemic lupus erythematosus, secondary syphilis, sickle cell anaemia.

19 (a) Angiokeratoma corporis diffusum (Anderson-Fabry's disease).
(b) Deficiency of ceramide galactosidase which leads to the deposition of glycolipid in the tissues and blood vessels.

20 (a) Varicella (chicken pox).
(b) Secondary infection, thrombocytopenic purpura, encephalitis, varicella pneumonia (usually in adults and those with an impaired immune response).

21 (a) A Kerion, i.e. an inflammatory form of tinea capitis – usually caused by *Trichophyton verrucosum* or *Trichophyton mentagrophytes*.
(b) With oral griseofulvin, taken until the fungus is no longer demonstrable.

22 (a) The patient underwent 'cupping' as a child for a pyrexial illness. This is post-inflammatory hyperpigmentation as a result of local 'burns'.
(b) Topical hydroquinone is often helpful.

23 (a) Xanthoma tuberosum.
(b) Coronary artery disease and occlusive peripheral arterial disease are common associations. This type of xanthoma is usually seen in Fredrickson, types II and III, hyperlipidaemias.

24 (a) Atopic dermatitis.
(b) Phenylketonuria; Wiskott-Aldrich syndrome; ataxia telangiectasia; Swiss-type agammaglobulinaemia.

25 (a) Cutaneous horn.
(b) Horny outgrowths may occur in or as a result of an underlying naevus, virus wart, keratoacanthoma, seborrhoeic keratosis or epidermoid cyst.
(c) Squamous cell carcinoma may develop in long established lesions which form in relatively normal skin.

26 (a) Morphoea (localised scleroderma).
(b) The natural history of the disease is towards spontaneous resolution.

27 (a) Habit-tic caused by the patient picking at the cuticles.
(b) Beau's lines – single transverse depression on the nails due to temporary interference with nail formation as a result of severe disease e.g. myocardial infarction, mumps or pneumonia.

28 (a) Pigmentation at the tip of the finger and loss of the nail.
(b) Malignant melanoma.

29 (a) Insulin induced fat hypertrophy.
(b) Local reactions: immediate or delayed erythema, keloid formation. General reactions: erythema multiforme, urticaria, purpura.

30 (a) Kaposi's varicelliform eruption (eczema herpeticum) in a child with atopic dermatitis.
(b) Infection with herpes simplex virus.
(c) The infection, usually primary, may cause encephalitis or dendritic ulceration of the cornea.

31 (a) Acanthosis nigricans.
(b) Mouth lesions; lesions over the palms (tripe hands) or soles; loss of weight or other evidence of malignancy.
(c) Malignancy of an internal organ occurs in almost 100 per cent of cases of the acquired type in non-obese adults. The cancers are commonly adenocarcinomas, 85 per cent being intra-abdominal.

32 (a) Neurofibromatosis.
(b) *Café-au-lait* patches, neurofibromata, pigmented hairy naevi, malignant degeneration of a neurofibroma (sarcoma formation 3–12%), neurogenic tumours – bilateral acoustic neuromata believed to occur almost exclusively in neurofibromatosis, epilepsy, kyphoscoliosis, associated endocrine disorders – acromegaly, Addison's disease or phaeochromocytoma.

33, 34 (a) Squamous cell carcinoma.
(b) Chondrodermatitis nodularis helicis; solar keratosis; basal cell carcinoma.

35 (a) Dilatation of the nail fold capillaries.
(b) May occur in systemic lupus erythematosus; systemic sclerosis; dermatomyositis.

36 (a) Pigmented seborrhoeic keratoses.
(b) Commonly acquired as a familial trait with no potential of malignant change within the tumours. A profuse eruption of seborrhoeic keratoses very occasionally may herald an internal malignant neoplasm.

37 (a) Metastases from a malignant melanoma.
(b) Sunlight; racial susceptibility; penetrating trauma or thermal injury to normal skin occasionally has given rise to a malignant melanoma.

38 (a) Erysipelas.
(b) General susceptibility is increased by malnutrition, alcoholism, undiagnosed diabetes mellitus, recent infections and dysgammaglobulinaemias. Predisposing local factors are oedema of renal or lymphatic origin.

39 (a) Gouty tophi.
(b) Renal colic from urate stones.

40 (a) Keratoacanthoma – the most frequently affected area is the central part of the face.
(b) Squamous cell carcinoma.

41, 42 (a) Fungal infection of the skin.
(b) Fungal hyphae and spores.

43 (a) Photosensitivity due to erythropoietic protoporphyria. The history of burning shortly after exposure to light and pock-like scarring are typical.
(b) Examination of peripheral blood for protoporphyrins.

44, 45, 46 (a) Tuberous sclerosis with adenoma sebaceum, periungual fibromas and hypopigmented leaf-shaped macules.
(b) Shagreen patches; intra-oral fibromas; *café-au-lait* patches; poliosis (60 per cent).

47, 48 (a) Basal cell carcinoma.
(b) Skin damaged by sunlight or irradiation; burn scars; vaccination scars; arsenic salts previously used as therapy for a variety of conditions, including psoriasis and as a 'tonic'.
(c) Invasion of the dermis with strands of deeply basophilic tumour cells.

49 (a) Cutaneous leishmaniasis.
(b) Transmitted by the sandfly, usually *Phlebotomus papatasii.*

50 (a) Infantile acne.
(b) Exceptionally, acne in infancy may be a manifestation of sexual precocity or a virilising syndrome.

51 (a) Ehlers-Danlos syndrome.
(b) Hyperelasticity of the skin, hyperextensible joints, ocular and internal manifestations, the latter dependent upon the Type of Ehlers-Danlos diagnosed. To date, 8 different varieties have been described.

52 (a) Psoriasis. The patient cut off the onycholytic distal edge of the nail.
(b) Pitting, onycholysis, subungual hyperkeratosis.

53 (a) Perioral dermatitis.
(b) Prolonged topical therapy with fluorinated steroids for usually a mild skin condition in the perinasal or perioral areas.

54, 55 (a) Chronic discoid lupus erythematosus.
(b) Skin biopsy.
(c) The inflammatory component responds well to treatment but scarring will remain, it is rare for this form to be associated with overt systemic lupus erythematosus.
(d) Hyperkeratosis and follicular plugging; epidermal atrophy; dense peri-appendageal lymphocytic infiltrate.

56 (a) The Hess or Rumpel-Leede (tourniquet) test.
(b) A sphygmomanometer cuff is applied to the upper arm as when the blood pressure is taken. It is then inflated to a pressure between diastolic and systolic which is maintained for 5 minutes. The cuff is deflated and the arm allowed to rest for 10 minutes, when the number of petechiae in a circumscribed area below the cuff is counted.
(c) Positive in diseases with increased capillary fragility; negative in coagulation disorders.

57 (a) Acute candidiasis.
(b) Diabetes mellitus, hypothyroidism, hypoparathyroidism drugs eg contraceptive pill, antibiotic therapy, systemic steroids.

58 (a) The Yellow-Nail syndrome.
(b) Recurrent pleural effusions, chronic bronchitis, bronchiectasis and lymphoedema usually of the lower limbs.
(c) Prolonged tetracycline therapy, eg for chest infections, very occasionally may cause a yellow discoloration of nails.

59 (a) Multiple halo naevi. The halo of depigmentation surrounds a pigmented naevus visible in the centre of many of the lesions.
(b) Halo naevi occur more commonly with vitiligo and, like vitiligo, occur more frequently with auto-immune disorders. Multiple halo naevi may occur also in patients with malignant melanoma.

60 (a) Lichen planus of the buccal mucosa.
(b) Focal keratosis or non-dyskeratotic leukoplakia – as a result of chronic irritation from jagged teeth, gum-biting or ill-fitting bridges; dyskeratotic leukoplakia; candidiasis; aphthous stomatitis; squamous papilloma; verruca vulgaris; secondary syphilis.

61 (a) Porphyria cutanea tarda. Patients exhibit photosensitivity with blister formation. The milia and scars form at sites of previous sub-epidermal bullae.
(d) Diabetes mellitus.

62 (a) Scrofuloderma (cutaneous tuberculosis).
(b) From the breakdown of skin overlying a tuberculous focus – in this case an infected joint.

63 (a) Erythema ab igne – seen most often on the legs of elderly women who sit close to gas or electric fires.
(b) Hypothyroidism.
(c) Epitheliomas may develop in keratoses which form in the later stages of the condition.

64 (a) Thyroid acropachy with periosteal new bone formation.
(b) Clubbing of the fingers, exophthalmos, pretibial myxoedema and other signs of thyrotoxicosis.

65 (a) 'Borderline' leprosy.
(b) Anhidrosis and anaesthesia over the plaques.
(c) Skin smear and skin biopsy.

66 (a) Rubber dermatitis from the elastic waist band in his pyjama trousers.
(b) Patch tests to rubber chemicals.

67 (a) Granuloma annulare.
(b) The majority of lesions clear spontaneously within 2 years.

68, 69, 70 (a) Candida infection; seborrhoeic dermatitis; Kaposi's sarcoma.
(b) Acquired immune deficiency syndrome (AIDS).
(c) He was homosexual.
(d) Folliculitis; recurrent fungal infection; vasculitis; herpes simplex; herpes zoster.

71 (a) Orf caused by a pox virus. Common in shepherds and veterinary surgeons.
(b) Recovery occurs spontaneously, usually within a month.

72 (a) Topical steroid-induced telangiectasia and atrophy. A fluorinated steroid was inappropriately applied for prolonged periods for infra-mammary psoriasis.

(b) Adrenal suppression specifically in children; steroid-induced rosacea; exacerbation of fungus and bacterial infections; increased intraocular pressure, open-angle glaucoma and cataracts from applications on the eye or use of steroid eye drops for long periods without remission. Cushing's syndrome from prolonged and extensive use in infants and young children.

73 (a) Eruptive xanthomata.
(b) Tendinous, tuberous and plane xanthomata.

74 (a) Bilateral ulnar paralysis leading to flattening of the hypothenar eminences and permanent flexion contracture of the ring and little fingers.
(b) Lepromatous leprosy.

75 (a) 'Strawberry' (angiomatous or cavernous) naevus.
(b) None – 90 per cent or more undergo complete or partial spontaneous resolution. Only 2–3 per cent fail completely to involute. Treatment then usually involves plastic surgery.

76 (a) Sarcoidosis.
(b) Vocal cord granuloma.
(c) Bilateral hilar lymphadenopathy.

77 (a) The 'butterfly' rash of systemic lupus erythematosus.
(b) Periungual erythema; nail fold telangiectasia; alopecia; livedo reticularis;

rticaria; purpura; hyperpigmentation; scarring eruption of discoid lupus
rythematosus.
c) Polyarthralgia or arthritis; pleurisy with or without effusion; pericarditis,
Libman-Sacks endocarditis; splenomegaly; localised or generalised lymphadenopathy; lupus nephritis. neurologic manifestations; retinal lesions – cotton wool
spots.

8 (a) Cutaneous tuberculosis.
b) 5 patterns are described and depend upon the local tissue response to infection
plaque-form, ulcerative, vegetative, tumour-like, papulo-nodular forms.
c) Squamous cell and less commonly basal cell carcinoma within the diseased
skin.

9 (a) Transverse ridge within the nodule differentiates it from a basal cell
carcinoma and confirms the diagnosis of granuloma fissuratum.
b) Ill-fitting spectacle frames which continually rub against the skin to produce the
tumour'. Histologically, lesions of long duration show granulomatous changes with
plasma cells.

10 (a) Tuberculoid leprosy.
b) Absence of hairs over the plaque, reduction or absence of sensation within the
plaque, eye lesions secondary to corneal anaesthesia.
c) Ulnar, common peroneal, great auricular and cervical nerves and the superficial
radial.

11 (a) Incontinentia pigmenti.
b) Dental – dentition may be delayed, peg shaped teeth may occur; ocular –
strabismus, optic atrophy. cataracts; CNS defects – mental retardation, epilepsy;
skeletal.

12 (a) White nails of cirrhosis. The colour change is thought to be in the nail bed
and not in the nail plate.
b) Clubbing; koilonychia – hypochromic anaemia; splinter haemorrhages – SBE,
ichinosis, severe rheumatoid arthritis; thin brittle nails – impaired peripheral
circulation; half-and-half nails – uraemia; azure half moons – hepatolenticular
degeneration (Kinnear-Wilson disease).

13 (a) Herpes zoster.
b) Children who have not had chicken pox should be kept away until the crusts
have separated.
c) Cancer, leukaemia, lymphoma, X-ray therapy, spinal puncture, neurosurgery,
immunosuppressive therapy and local trauma.

14 (a) Fixed drug eruption.
b) Phenolphthalein found in some laxatives; sulphonamides, antimalarials,
chlordiazepoxide, oxyphenbutazone.

15 (a) Acne vulgaris.
b) Androgen associated seborrhoea; lipophilic anaerobic bacteria, *Propioni-
acterium acnes* within the pilosebaceous follicle; composition of sebum.
c) Acne has familial bias. In a survey one or both parents of half of the patients
had suffered from acne. Fewer than ten per cent of boys *without* acne had a parent
with a history of acne. Men with the XYY genotype are pre-disposed to nodulo-
cystic acne.

16 (a) Acute 'contact' dermatitis.
b) Ophthalmic medications, including antibiotics, atropine and mercurial pre-
parations; plants, especially Primula obconica in this patient; nickel dermatitis;
cosmetics, especially nail varnish.
c) Patch testing against suspected allergens.

87 (a) 'Lick' eczema as a result of constantly licking the lips – often a nervous tic.
(b) Perioral dermatitis, atopic dermatitis.

88 (a) Seborrhoeic dermatitis.
(b) In the flexures, axillae, groins, anogenital and submammary regions. Presternal and interscapular areas are particularly commonly affected in men.
(c) Psoriasis; contact dermatitis; pemphigus erythematosus; in the flexures, candidiasis, dermatophyte infections and erythrasma.

89 (a) Xanthelasmata.
(b) Essential familial hypercholesterolaemia; primary biliary cirrhosis; diabetes mellitus; usually no underlying cause is found.
(c) By cautery or trichloracetic acid or excision.

90 (a) Chronic radiodermatitis.
(b) Decreased pigmentation, decreased sebaceous activity, skin atrophy, hair loss, radionecrotic ulceration, underlying bone sequestration, basal cell epithelioma, post-radiation sarcoma.

91, 92 (a) Lichen simplex exacerbated by constant scratching. She was prescribed topical steroid therapy for a fortnight.
(b) There is no destruction of skin or of the nipple.

93 (a) Epidermoid cysts.
(b) Calcification of the contents of epidermoid cysts situated on the chest may appear as opacities on chest X-ray.

94 (a) Dermatosis papulosa nigra. The lesions are naevoid developmental defects of pilosebaceous follicles.
(b) The lesions are benign, non-infectious but gradually increase in number. They must be differentiated from viral warts and seborrhoeic keratoses.

95 (a) Linear pigmented naevus. Very common in coloured people, for whom it is usually of no significance.
(b) A single dark band in a nail of a white person also indicates a junctional naevus in the matrix. The importance lies in the potential of such lesions becoming malignant melanomas.

96 (a) Peutz-Jeghers syndrome.
(b) Malignant degeneration of an intestinal polyp.

97, 98 (a) Lesions of molluscum contagiosum.
(b) A pox virus.
(c) All children who have not previously had them, particularly those with atopic dermatitis, and immunosuppressed adults.
(d) Accumulations of darkly staining molluscum bodies within the epidermis. Molluscum bodies are enlarged damaged epidermal cells containing the virus.

99 (a) Discoid lupus erythematosus.
(b) Lichen planus, sarcoid, cicatricial pemphigoid, congenital scalp defects, some congenital naevi, folliculitis decalvans, radiotherapy, scleroderma and occasionally following ringworm kerion and herpes zoster infection of the scalp.

100 (a) Systemic sclerosis. He shows the typical 'pinched' appearance of the nose and blotchy telangiectasia.
(b) Dilated nail fold capillaries; finger pulp atrophy; beaking of the nails (pseudo-clubbing); pigmentation of the skin; calcinosis cutis; hepatomegaly; myopathy; hypertension and its sequelae.

101 (a) Hand, foot and mouth disease.
(b) On the feet, in the mouth, sometimes also on the buttocks.
(c) Coxsackie virus A16.
(d) Throat swab and faeces examined for the organism.

102 (a) Cauliflower ear.
(b) He was a (not very successful) professional boxer.
(c) Repeated trauma with recurrent oedema, haemorrhage and fibrosis.

103 (a) Erosive lichen planus.
(b) Pemphigus vulgaris, recurrent aphthae, Behçet's disease, Stevens-Johnson syndrome, recurrent herpes simplex.

104 (a) Alopecia areata.
(b) In most patients patches regrow completely in a few months, some follow a relapsing pattern and in some cases all the hair is lost (alopecia totalis).
(c) Ringworm infection (tinea capitis), hair plucking.

105 (a) Atopic dermatitis.
(b) Face and neck, elbow, wrist and ankle flexures.
(c) Asthma, hay fever, migraine, cataracts, susceptibility to drug reactions and to topical viral infections.

106 (a) A superficial basal cell carcinoma.
(b) It is often associated with previous excessive sun exposure, or X-ray treatment, of the area. If the basal cell carcinoma forms on skin protected from light, any previous contact or medication with arsenic in earlier life should be investigated.
(c) By curettage, cryotherapy or excision.
(d) Bowen's disease (intraepidermal carcinoma).

107 (a) Darier's disease (Keratosis follicularis).
(b) Autosomal dominant.
(c) Small stature, low intelligence, low fertility in women; rarely diffuse pulmonary fibrosis (lower zone) with nodulation, bone cysts.

108 (a) A dental sinus and granuloma, due to an infected root.
(b) X-ray of the jaws to display the apices of the teeth.
(c) Surgical extraction of the tooth, or residual root, responsible.

109, 110 (a) A symmetrical patchy purplish-red (heliotrope) erythema over the face (including the upper eyelids), and over the knuckles with streaks of erythema along the extensor surfaces of the fingers extending to the nail folds.
(b) Muscle weakness and arthritis.
(c) Dermatomyositis.
(d) A malignant neoplasm in a significant number of patients over 40 years old.

111 (a) Artefacts.
(b) Pyoderma gangrenosum, cicatricial pemphigoid, arteritic ulcers, various infective or neoplastic ulcers (skin biopsy often helps to distinguish the correct diagnosis).
(c) Lesions may continue for many years, with or without topical or psychological treatment.

112 (a) Erythema nodosum.
(b) Sarcoidosis, post-streptococcal infection, drug-associated (e.g. sulphonamides), primary tuberculosis, Behçet's disease, ulcerative colitis, lymphogranuloma venereum, cat-scratch disease, blastomycosis, coccidioidomycosis, yersinia (pasteurella) infections, lymphoma. In many cases no cause is found.

113 (a) The simple dominant form of epidermolysis bullosa. Several severe dystrophic forms of the disorder occur, with either dominant or recessive inheritance.
(b) Recurrent podopompholyx (eczema).

114 (a) Tinea pedis.
(b) Microscopic examination and culture of skin scrapings to demonstrate and identify the fungus.

115 (a) Infectious mononucleosis with exanthem. An eruption almost invariably occurs in this condition if the patient has been treated with ampicillin.
(b) Palatal petechiae, enlarged spleen.

116 (a) Urticaria pigmentosa (cutaneous mastocytosis).
(b) In the bones (lucencies and opacities are seen on bone X-ray).
(c) All the lesions tend to clear after a number of years.

117 (a) Keloid scars.
(b) Burns, skin infections, skin trauma of any kind.
(c) Pruritus is common in large keloids, occasionally pain.
(d) They usually recur larger than before.

118 (a) Leukaemic infiltration of the skin.
(b) Acute myelo-monocytic leukaemia, which is the commonest of the leukaemias to give rise to skin nodules.

119 (a) The drug used to treat her urinary infection, nalidixic acid, had photo-sensitised her skin and the sun exposure caused the blisters. The areas covered by her shoes and trousers were unaffected.
(b) Systemic lupus erythematosus; rosacea; porphyria cutanea tarda.

120 (a) Congenital pigmented melanocytic naevus.
(b) Spina bifida.
(c) Some of these lesions, usually the large ones, develop malignant melanoma.

121 (a) Mycosis fungoides, a T-cell lymphoma initially confined to the skin.
(b) Skin biopsy.
(c) Slow extension of skin lesions with eventual tumour formation and systemic dissemination of lymphoma. In most patients this process takes several decades.

122 (a) Oculocutaneous albinism.
(b) It is autosomal recessive, often with a history of consanguinity in the previous generation.
(c) In order to treat eye problems, and to detect and treat skin tumours in sun-exposed areas e.g. actinic keratoses, basal and squamous carcinomas and malignant melanomas.

123 (a) Pityriasis rosea.
(b) A 'herald patch' which is similar, but usually of larger size than the lesions shown.
(c) It usually clears six weeks after the onset of the widespread eruption.

124 (a) He has pityriasis versicolor. A chronic and relapsing yeast infection caused by the organism *Malassezia furfur*. This produces azalaic acid which bleaches melanin.
(b) It is not to be confused with vitiligo where there is usually total loss of skin melanin in affected areas.

125 (a) It is a port-wine naevus.
(b) It can be part of the Sturge-Weber syndrome which comprises skin, eye and brain angiomas. Neurological defects include epilepsy, hemiplegia and mental retardation.

126 (a) Pseudoxanthoma elasticum.
(b) Sides of the neck, axillae, periumbilical area and groins.
(c) Vascular wall degeneration in the gut can lead to recurrent haemorrhages.
(d) Retinal degeneration (with the finding of angioid streaks), hypertension, angina, cerebral haemorrhage, intermittent claudication.

127 (a) Anogenital psoriasis.
(b) The possibility of fungal and candida infection can be excluded by microscopic examination of skin scrapings.

128 (a) Amyloid: in this case secondary to multiple myeloma.

129 (a) Rosacea. the features are erythema, oedema, papules, pustules and telangiectasia.
(b) Flushing and blushing, sore eyes (due to rosacea keratoconjunctivitis).
(c) Daily low dose of wide-spectrum antibiotic for about 4 months in the first instance.

130 (a) Relapsing polychondritis; the ear lobe which does not contain cartilage is spared.
(b) Skin biopsy shows cartilage which is damaged and surrounded by lymphocytes; during attacks there is increased urinary acid mucopolysaccharide excretion.
(c) In nasal, joint, laryngeal, tracheal, bronchial and costal cartilages.

131 (a) Sarcoidosis.
(b) Soft tissue swellings and bone cysts.

132 (a) Lupus pernio (sarcoidosis).
(b) Rhinophyma, lupus vulgaris, leprosy.

133 (a) A body louse (*Pediculus humanus corporis*).
(b) Pruritus with weals, papules, erythema and eczema.
(c) In seams, hems and folds of clothing, rarely on the skin surface.
(d) Topical therapy with an insecticide (e.g. gamma benzene hexachloride) for patients and contacts, with auto-claving of clothing.

134 Striae caused by excessive use of potent topical corticosteroids in an adolescent girl with atopic dermatitis.

135 (a) Squamous carcinoma.
(b) Biopsy for histopathology.
(c) Excessive sunlight exposure.

136 (a) Secondary syphilis.
(b) TPHA (treponema pallidum haemagglutination test) and VDRL.

137 (a) Tinea capitis (scalp ringworm).
(b) Microscopic examination and culture of hairs at the margins of the patches to demonstrate fungus; Wood's light examination of the scalp (infected hairs often fluoresce).
(c) Oral griseofulvin, taken until the fungus can no longer be demonstrated on microscopy of hairs.

138 (a) Lesions of Kaposi's sarcoma.
(b) Middle aged-elderly patients, often of eastern Mediterranean origin; young patients with acquired immunodeficiency syndrome secondary to infection with the HTLV–III virus.
(c) Pigmentation associated with stasis dermatitis.
(d) Good in the elderly, poor in the young.

139 (a) Tinea unguium (ringworm fungal infection of the nails).
(b) Nails clippings examined microscopically and cultured to detect and identify the fungus.
(c) The thickened nail is more susceptible to minor trauma in the shoe.

140 (a) Urticaria.
(b) Acute (e.g. related to foods and drugs); physical (e.g. heat, cold, pressure, solar, cholinergic, aquagenic) and chronic. It is uncommonly related to systemic disease (e.g. S.L.E. or gut infestations).
(c) With oral antihistamines in sufficient dose and frequency to control the pruritus and lesions.

141 (a) They have arisen in acne scars.
(b) Intralesional steroid injections can be helpful but improvement is slow and often incomplete.

142, 143, 144 (a) Scabies.
(b) Excoriations due to generalised pruritus; a burrow in a finger web; the acarus of *Sarcoptes scabiei* var. *hominis*, which has been scraped out of a burrow.
(c) By close physical contact with an infested person. Pruritus starts about six weeks after the disease is first acquired; with subsequent infections the incubation period is considerably shortened.
(d) By two applications of an anti-scabetic lotion (benzyl benzoate or gammabenzene hexachloride) to the whole skin surface below the chin, on two occasions 24 hours apart for patient and close contacts. Pruritus can take up to two weeks to settle, during which time no further anti-scabetic treatment should be used.

145 (a) Secondary syphilis.
(b) Palms and trunk, erythematous and brownish macules and papules at all stages of evolution, glistening 'snail-track' erosions in mouth, papular flat warts (condylomata lata) in perianal region.

146 (a) Vitiligo.
(b) Diabetes mellitus, Addison's disease, thyroid disease (both hyper- and hypo-thyroidism) and pernicious anaemia.
(c) Yes; contact with chemicals such as catechols, phenols and hydroquinones.
(d) Vogt-Koyanagi-Harada syndrome.

147 (a) Degos' disease (malignant atrophic papulosis).
(b) Lesions in the gut may lead to fatal haemorrhage and perforation. Neurological signs can result from central nervous system lesions.

148 (a) Micropapular sarcoid; this pattern is commoner in black people.
(b) Acne vulgaris; acne rosacea; acne agminata; adenoma sebaceum; secondary syphilis; insect bites; varicella; tuberculosis; milia; viral warts; syringomas; trio-choepitheliomas; basal cell naevus syndrome; folliculitis.

149 (a) Gonococcal septicaemia.
(b) Repeated blood cultures on media suitable for growing the gonococcus are required; swabs from the skin lesions rarely grow the organism but it may be detectable by a fluorescent antibody technique.

150, 151 (a) A bed bug (*Cimex lenticularis*).
(b) It is heat seeking.

152 (a) Pityriasis versicolor. The eruption can manifest itself either as pink or brownish patches on a pale background, or as hypopigmented patches on a dark background (hence 'versicolor').
(b) The yeast *Malassezia furfur*.
(c) With topical agents e.g. benzoic acid compound ointment BPC (Whitfield's ointment), selenium sulphide lotion, creams or lotions of the imidazole group. None offers a permanent cure.

153 (a) Traction, in this case due to repeated use of tight metal curlers. Other possible causes are 'pulled-back' hair styles, hair straightening tongs and neurotic picking of the hair.
(b) If the traction is stopped, some, but not all, of the hairs will regrow.

154 (a) Bazin's disease (erythema induratum), a cutaneous manifestation of tuberculosis in an individual with strong delayed hypersensitivity to tubercular antigen.
(b) Screening of lungs, gut, renal and genital tracts for active tuberculosis; however, in Bazin's disease often no active focus is detectable.
(c) With a full course of systemic antituberculous drugs.

155 (a) He has pediculosis (phthiriasis) pubis. A 'crab louse' is just to the right of centre, and refractile eggs (nits) are attached to the eyelashes.
(b) In pubic hair but infestation of axillary, moustache and eyelid hairs is not uncommon; the diagnosis is easily missed if eggs and lice are present in small numbers.

156 (a) Fish tank granulomas.
(b) Keeping tropical fish.
(c) *Mycobacterium marinum*.
(d) Swimming pool granuloma (same organism), sporotrichosis, lupus vulgaris, leishmaniasis.

157 The arterial supply to the hallux is impaired, leading to ischaemia and incipient or actual gangrene. A relatively common cause is arterio-sclerosis secondary to diabetes but a similar appearance can occur in embolism, polyarteritis nodosa, thrombo-angiitis obliterans (Buerger's disease) and ergot intoxication.

158 (a) Generalised pustular psoriasis (von Zumbusch). It usually arises in patients with a history of psoriasis which has become unstable, sometimes as a reaction to inappropriate topical or systemic treatment.
(b) Toxic epidermal necrolysis.
(c) With systemic methotrexate in small doses.

159 (a) Porphyria cutanea tarda.
(b) Alcohol or other hepatotoxic chemicals.
(c) Raised urinary uroporphyrin and faecal coproporphyrin.

160 (a) Cold urticaria. There is a familial form (dominant inheritance) and an acquired form. In both there is pruritic weating in response to chilling of the skin. Sudden immersion in cold water can lead to unconsciousness or even death and patients should be warned of this. Unfortunately, the 'ice cube test' is not always positive in patients with typical symptoms of the complaint.

(b) Raynaud's phenomenon; perniosis (chilblains); erythromelalgia; cold panniculitis; cryoglobulinaemia.

161 (a) He had acquired a *Pseudomonas pyocyanea* septicaemia.

(b) Leukaemic infiltration and nodules (leukaemia cutis); chloroma; erythroderma.

162 (a) The Koebner (or isomorphic) phenomenon.

(b) Psoriasis; vitiligo; warts and molluscum contagiosum.

163 (a) Livedo reticularis.

(b) It is an abnormal vascular pattern which may be congenital or 'idiopathic', or associated with arterial disease, 'collagen diseases', or with chronic infections and malignant disease.

164 She has psoriasis (note finger-nail dystrophy) with psoriatic arthritis mutilans. In this severe form of arthritis there is subluxation of joints with osteolysis and eventual ankylosis.

165 Adolescent striae. They are particularly related to the growth spurt in adolescence but similar lesions can occur later in life, associated with rapid weight gain or loss.

166 (a) Impetigo contagiosa.

(b) Either *Staphylococcus aureus* or *Streptococcus pyogenes*.

(c) Acute glomerulonephritis, if the skin was infected by a nephritogenic streptococcus.

167 (a) Frontoparietal morphoea, or morphoea 'en coup de sabre' (i.e. resembling a scar from a sabre cut).

(b) It could extend downwards and more deeply to produce atrophy of all the tissues down to and including bone, with facial asymmetry and malalignment of teeth and jaw.

(c) Ocular problems occur if the line of the lesion passes through the eye; there can be electro-encephalogram abnormalities below an area of affected skull.

168 (a) He has actinic dermatitis (photosensitive eczema) and his clothing has protected his skin from the effects of the light.

(b) Drugs of the tetracycline, thiazide, phenothiazide, sulphonamide and sulphonylurea groups, either topically or systemically, can be photosensitising.

169 (a) Nodules of calcinosis cutis.

(b) Systemic sclerosis, dermatomyositis, abnormalities of parathyroid function, hypervitaminosis D, the milk-alkali syndrome and metastatic bone disease. Sometimes no cause is found.

170 (a) Dermatitis herpetiformis.

(b) Gluten enteropathy (coeliac disease).

(c) On the scalp, face, neck, sacral area and knees.

(d) Scabies.

(e) With dapsone tablets and a gluten-free diet.

171 (a) Haemochromatosis (this condition is only rarely seen in women).
b) Skin biopsy frequently, and liver biopsy regularly, demonstrate excessive iron deposition.
c) Addison's disease, chronic renal failure, porphyria cutanea tarda, thyrotoxicosis, ectopic ACTH syndrome, primary biliary cirrhosis and, rarely, ochronosis.

172 (a) Erythrasma, an infection with the diphtheroid *Corynebacterium minutissimum*.
b) Diabetes mellitus.
c) Skin scrapings show masses of tiny bacteria microscopically: Wood's light (filtered ultraviolet light) shone on the skin shows coral pink fluorescence in affected areas (the bacteria produce porphyrins which account for the fluorescence).

173 (a) He has recessively inherited ichthyosis vulgaris of the sex-linked type, which is darker than the much commoner dominant ichthyosis vulgaris and much less likely to improve with age.
b) Lymphoma; myeloma; sarcoid.

174 (a) Bowen's disease (intra-epidermal carcinoma).
b) Basal cell carcinoma, psoriasis, actinic keratosis.
c) They grow larger, often ulcerate and occasionally develop into invasive squamous cell carcinoma.

175 (a) He has a black hairy tongue (the degree of 'hairiness' is variable) due to hyperplasia of filiform papillae.
b) Systemic and topical antibiotics, excessive smoking. Often no cause is apparent.

176 (a) Pityriasis alba (a form of eczema).
b) It usually clears during, or before, adolescence.

177 (a) Photo-onycholysis, related to hot sun exposure.
b) Most cases are related to taking photosensitising drugs, such as demethylchlor-tetracycline.

178 (a) They are bullous insect bite reactions, probably from cat or dog fleas.
b) Contact with dogs or cats or walking in a garden or rural area in the Summer predisposes to these lesions. The intensity of the reaction is a host response and most individuals develop pruritic papules without blistering. Blistering reactions are common in children.

179 (a) Candida intertrigo ('erosio interdigitale blastomycetica').
b) Persistent wetness of the finger webs, occupational or otherwise. Deformity of the fingers (e.g. in rheumatoid arthritis) make it more likely to appear.

180 (a) Henoch-Schönlein purpura.
b) Bleeding from the gut and nephritis.
c) Usually none is found. In former years streptococcal infection was thought to be important. It is now regarded as an immune complex disease but the antigen is usually difficult to identify.

181 (a) Larva migrans ('creeping eruption').
b) Larvae of various hookworms and tapeworms which usually infest dogs and cats. The larvae penetrate the skin of the host on a beach or other contaminated area.
c) Occasionally pulmonary eosinophilia (Loeffler's syndrome) is seen with larva migrans.
d) The larva eventually dies after a number of weeks or months because it is in the wrong host. More rapid resolution can be obtained by topical application of thiabendazole or of liquid nitrogen.

182 (a) Chloasma. The cheeks and upper lip are often affected also.
(b) It is both sunlight and hormone dependent. It occurs commonly during and after pregnancy or as a result of taking the oral contraceptive pill.

183 (a) She had been prescribed a potent topical corticosteroid cream for mild acne spots, and then developed erythema and pustules as a result of the prolonged topical steroid therapy.
(b) Stop the topical steroid application. A prolonged course of oral low-dose tetracycline therapy (three months or more) usually improves the condition.

184 (a) 'Tripe' palms.
(b) Acanthosis nigricans.
(c) Rugose thickening and pigmentation of the axillae and anogenital region, scattered warty lesions.
(d) The adult form is nearly always associated with a malignant neoplasm.

185 (a) Chronic mucocutaneous candidiasis.
(b) The diagnosis encompasses several genetic syndromes in which are found defects of delayed hypersensitivity, low serum iron and endocrine deficiencies (e.g. parathyroid, thyroid, adrenal and anterior pituitary).

186 (a) Psoriasis vulgaris.
(b) Scalp, nails, knees, umbilicus, lower back and anogenital area.
(c) Various forms of arthropathy: rheumatoid arthritis-like; osteo-arthritis-like, affecting distal interphalangeal joints of the fingers; ankylosing spondylitis-like, affecting sacro-iliac joints; arthritis mutilans.

Index

Numbers refer to illustrations

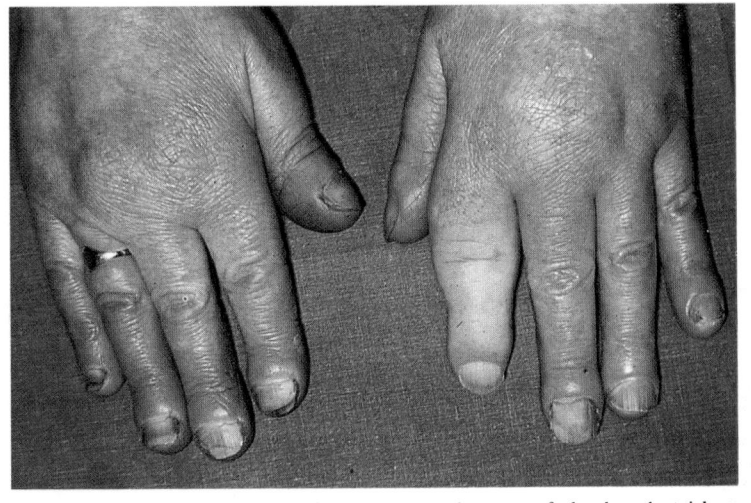

64 Diffuse soft tissue thickening over the dorsum of the hands with marked bony swelling of the left index finger.
(a) What is the condition?
(b) What other physical signs should you look for?

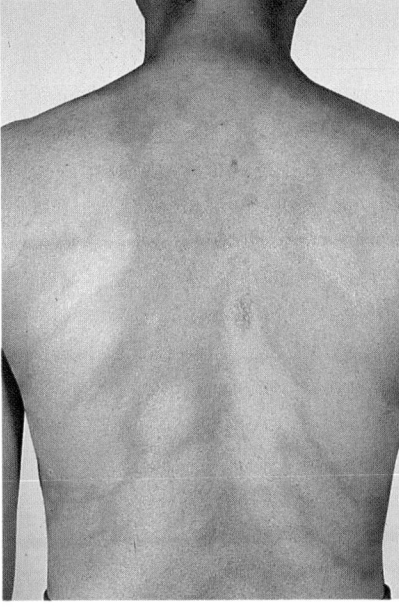

65 Multiple hypopigmented plaques distributed asymmetrically over the back. Many of the plaques showed hair loss.
(a) What condition should be suspected?
(b) What other physical signs would aid in diagnosis?
(c) How would you confirm the clinical suspicion?

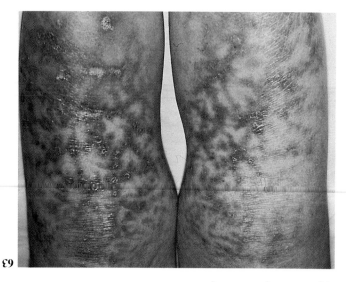

62 A slow growing ulcer over the dorsum of the foot. Biopsy showed no malignancy but suggested a diagnosis which was confirmed on culture of tissue.
(a) What was the diagnosis?
(b) How does it result?

63 This condition is frequently associated with cold weather.
(a) What is it?
(b) What may it signal?
(c) How may it be complicated?

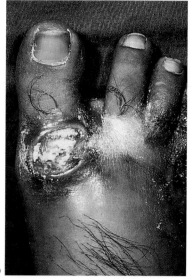